HELL STARTED AT 24

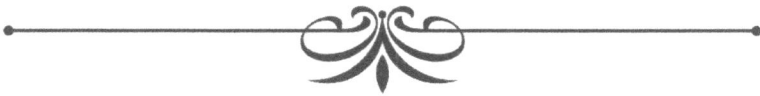

By
Kettlyne StCyr, MSN, APRN, PMHNP
and Jupshy Jasmin, RN, MSN

ISBN-13: 978-1-7370632-0-9

Untold Secret Beauty Publishing

Printed in the United States of America

Acknowledgment

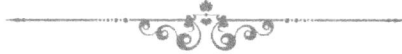

I would love to thank my children, family, and friends for all their

support.

Jose Luis Medina, a special thank you for all selfless collaborations

and loyalty.

Contents

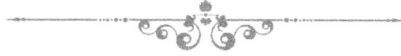

Introduction
Peace Before the Storm

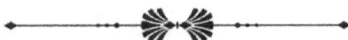

It was a beautiful winter day, warm and dry in South Florida. I was glad to be off from work so that I could run my errands. My first stop would be the bank, then the dry cleaner, hardware store, maybe take my mother to lunch, and end with the supermarket. This evening, I was planning a delicious meal for my family.

I had a beautiful home, a loving husband, a precious son, and Christmas was not too far off. I was in my early twenties and blessed with good health. At work, I had received recognition for being a hardworking employee. And amongst my circle of friends, I was known for being generous, caring, and dependable. In fact, all those qualities made me the gal who was always willing to lend a helping hand. After all, when one is fortunate, why not help those who need a leg up or a push in the right direction?

I was grateful for what I had, and I did not take it for granted. The casual observer would say I had it all. And even though life was not perfect, it was pretty darn good. I had so much to live for. I was living the American Dream!

A little after mid-day, I began to experience a growing uneasiness. First, my heart raced, then slowed back to normal. Then, the episode repeated again, then once more. I was frightened and questioning my health as I tried to recall my last medical check-up.

Above me, the sky darkened. The swirls and curls of fluffy white clouds were pushed aside by a restless march of angry rainclouds that quickly spread from one horizon to the other. The sun was swallowed up, vanishing from the sky…except for a tiny sliver of light piercing the gloom. Could it be enough to dispel the ocean of blackness and illuminate the world once more?

I watched the lone ray of brightness and hope struggle valiantly against the vastness, and I was tempted to cheer aloud for it to triumph. It was as if the heavens were sending a positive message to me. But the shadows were not defeated yet. The wind blew, and rain brought the crackling sound of thunder. A blinding flash of light followed, signaling that the time of judgment and destruction had arrived. Twilight was upon us!

I found myself running, dodging bolts of lightning that struck the earth near me, splashing gaseous fire and blinding me, deafening me. As the storm grew in intensity, each lightning strike got closer and closer. I was knocked down, my hands and knees bloodied, but I found the strength to rise and go on.

This cannot be real. It must be a nightmare, I thought. There was no refuge to be found. Then, in my path, I saw shelter: a lonely house. I rushed toward it only to find it burning to ashes and dust. On the ground was a garden hose. I reached for it, but my hand could not grasp it. The ground melted away as flames rose into the air around me.

I woke up breathless, drenched in sweat, and in significant physical and emotional discomfort. It felt as if I had just journeyed deep into Hell and somehow survived it.

Was it a mere nightmare or a prophetic dream?

We never really think these things through too much. Do we? These brief glimpses of Hell that sometimes haunt our dreams?

We know Hell is supposed to be a hot and horrible place with a specific purpose, but as enlightened individuals, we never think about it any further. We never wonder about its existence because it lies outside of human sense perception. The glorious days of yore when mankind struggled to understand the mystical and the spiritual has faded. In the age of reason, we feed on rationalization and logic and fail to imagine and explore the possibilities that lie beyond tangible reality. Like Hell.

Humanity has too many REAL problems to worry about what cannot be seen or touched. We look both ways when crossing the street, even when the light is red. We put on our seat belts, we purchase life insurance, we maintain a healthy fear of heights and darkness and fire and storms. Some of us may pray in our beds each night. But we are not too concerned about Hell. Why bother thinking about it? Life is complicated and time-consuming. We are busy with all the good and bad of the human condition, of the daily grind. Why be fearful or anxious about Hell, something that cannot hurt us?

In hindsight, whether it was a prophetic omen or indigestion, I should have put more stock in that nightmare. I certainly did not think Hell would ever arrive at my doorstep. Things were going well for me. My existence was rewarding. I felt blessed. The important thing was that even though no relationship is perfect, my husband was at my side to assure me that I was loved and cherished. We had each other. I birthed a child from that love. A sweet, funny, curious, wonderful little human. His laughter was contagious, and it brought immeasurable happiness into my life.

My world was far from perfect, but it was good. It all felt eternal. I swore it would last a lifetime. I loved my life. But nothing that could have or should have delivered me into the depths of Hell...or so I thought.

Ten days before my twenty-fourth birthday, I was visited, quite literally, by the dove of destiny, the legendary incarnation of fate representative of the crossroads we all encounter at unexpected moments in our lives. On ivory-colored wings, the arrival of the little bird does not necessarily bring bad tidings. It can deliver the promise of both opportunity or danger. Balance or chaos. Crucial decisions must be made. One path may lead to peace of mind and fortune, while choosing a different direction may result in the kiss of flames that leave nothing but embers and ashes in its wake.

If only we could see the end result before committing to action. If only we knew what we could stand to gain or lose. Could there be clues, warnings, or signs that could protect an undeserving victim from brutal pitfalls? With the possibility of random and spontaneous events occurring all around us at any given time, many consider interpreting divine messages to be mere superstition. A shooting star, therefore, carries little significance to modern man.

We no longer look for hidden meanings in our environment. Perhaps we should. Not in nature but in other surroundings, in our work and home, in our circle of friends. Failing to recognize or acknowledge the obvious hints of trouble is what puts us in vulnerable situations.

My existence unraveled when I answered a cry for help. The day began like any other mundane day...cooking, housekeeping, laundry, no time for exercise. And then there was a phone call that put me at a crossroads. I did not hesitate to make the decision I believed to be right, a decision that most people would make given the circumstances. Destiny, however, had a detour in mind. And the script was laden with hardship and misery. It began with a spark that led to a fire and billowing smoke. As I stood before the inferno, looking at my personal apocalypse through the smoke and haze, I knew the fabled dove of my childhood, as white as freshly fallen snow, was flying over the ruin that was once my home. Untouched by the flames, it continued to circle higher and higher, gaining altitude until it reached the heavens. Despite feeling weak and shattered, I always imagined the presence of the dove, the symbol of hope and healing, to be nearby looking over me. Little did I know that this tragedy was only the beginning of a series of tests of perseverance. The worst was yet to come.

I invite readers into my story, into my life and world, into my distress and despair. In one single year, I suffered one challenging experience after another. Each incident was a crisis, and at every step, I questioned past and present life choices. Doubt, remorse, disability, isolation, and many other negative emotions and consequences threaded every fiber of my being. In my descent into what seemed like the very lowest depths of Hell, positivity and wondrous things were reintroduced into my life.

What happened to me can happen to anyone. My hope is to enlighten readers with an amplified awareness of mental health, an essential part of one's well-being.

Chapter 1
Suddenly My World Crashes

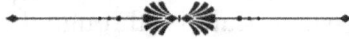

Ten days before my twenty-fourth birthday, a good friend suffered an episode of domestic abuse. In the middle of the night, the man she was living with took her clothes and belongings and threw them out of the house and into the front yard. When friends get into relationship disputes of this magnitude, I am the voice of reason who encourages them to walk away for the sake of their health and safety. In this situation, the woman had nowhere to go, and she had a four-year-old son with her. I did not have the heart to leave her out on the streets helpless and vulnerable with a preschooler in her care.

The solution was to get the woman and her son to safety as quickly as possible. Within the hour, I drove to her location, helped her pick up some belongings off the ground, and welcomed them into my home. What I did not know was that I was also inviting trouble. I was happy to help her in a time of great need. I refused to take money throughout her stay. She did not have to pay for food or boarding because I sympathized with her situation and felt it was the least I could do to help her get back on her feet. We perused the newspaper together in my free time, looking for employment opportunities she was qualified for. I wanted to provide my friend with every opportunity to embark on a safe and prosperous new life.

I felt secure knowing that although the man whom my friend was involved with knew me, he did not know where I lived. Nevertheless, the potential for danger was present. We devised a safety plan that involved calling 9-1-1 and getting herself and her son to safety. As the days went by, my friend seemed to be at peace with how the new chapter of her life was playing out. Her demeanor steadily improved even though job prospects did not pan out. Most importantly, she did not seem to be bothered by phantoms of her past. Before long, I stopped worrying about her.

As for me, with Christmas approaching fast, I took every opportunity to work extra shifts as an EMT technician in either of my two jobs. My routine after work was to pick up my three-year-old son from the babysitter and drive home. However, one evening, when I went to pick up my son, the babysitter asked for advice addressing a personal problem. She expressed it had nothing to do with childcare duties but needed to confide in someone she could trust. Needless to say, I was delayed.

After helping the babysitter resolve distressing issues that were bothering her, it was time to go home. On the way, another friend contacted me to discuss a personal situation she was going through. Although exhausted from working a long twenty-four-hour shift on an ambulance, I knew that she needed me, and I stopped by her house as well. As she explained her situation, I realized that it was not going to be a quick conversation. Consequently, I invited her to spend the night at my house so that I could unwind from work before continuing the conversation. She understood that I had worked a long shift and agreed to watch my son for me and spend the night. Rush hour traffic had long melted away, and the drive to my home was delightful.

On the horizon, miles from my destination, I saw heavy clouds of dark smoke in the direction I was heading. Something was obviously burning. Due to the volume, I thought it was surely a filling station or a factory spreading the black mushroom of darkness over my corner of the city. As I drove closer, I noticed the smoke was awfully close to where I lived and hoped we would not be burdened by toxic fumes. As I rounded the last corner, I discovered that the smoke that was flooding the neighborhood and rising into the sky was coming from my house.

MY HOUSE WAS ON FIRE!

The shock and disbelief I experienced at that moment threw me into a panic. My heart was racing so fast it almost burst out of my chest. My whole world stopped at that moment. It felt like time was at a standstill as I tried to wrap my head around what I saw. It was a nightmare, only I was not asleep. It was all too real.

Before long, like in any fire scene, there will be dozens of spectators and plenty of fire trucks, rescue vehicles, and police cars.

There was nowhere to park and so much commotion with people clogging the streets watching the horror unfold.

Pulling into the parking lot of a retail store about a quarter-mile away, I left my son in my friend's care and made my way back to the scene on foot. I had to push my way through the masses, trying to get to where I could ask someone in authority what had happened. I was very concerned about my other friend, the one who was staying with me. Could she or her son have been injured?

When I finally arrived at the barricade tape, I collapsed onto my knees. The police officers saw my reaction and asked if I was the owner or knew the owner.

I breathlessly gestured that I was the owner. One of the police officers asked for my husband by name. I told the officer my husband was at work, but a woman and child were inside. The information prompted a flurry of activity until word came back that no bodies were found in the home.

I was moved to the back of a rescue vehicle. The minor wounds I suffered from falling were treated, and I was given water. Police officers escorted my friend and my son to a nearby location. While they were there, I was able to convince my friend to take my son back to her house until I could join them. As tired as I was, I had to stick around and figure out what to do next.

My once beautiful home was now nothing more than a smoking lump of charcoal. Around midnight, when the fire was completely extinguished, and the embers had cooled, the house was deemed safe to enter. With flashlights in hand, a pair of crime scene investigators led me inside, room by room, to explain what happened. I had to agree not to touch anything until the investigation was completed. In the master bedroom, one of the investigators shared evidence that gasoline had been poured onto the bed before it was lit on fire. He asked if gasoline had been stored in the home. I informed him that a few cans of old paint may have been lying around, but no gasoline or anything combustible. As we continued to walk throughout the burned structure, the same man demonstrated how a device designed to identify chemicals used to accelerate fire was instrumental in collecting evidence.

The other crime scene investigator confided that if gasoline was brought into the home by the perpetrator, then this was a premeditated crime and not an impulsive act. He told me that if I had walked in at the wrong time, whoever did this could have just as easily turned the rage against me. By the grace of God, the delays I had experienced on the way home may have spared the lives of my son and me.

I contacted my husband to break the bad news to him. He asked me to stop kidding around and let him get back to work. It took a little persuasive convincing to assure him I was being truthful. I think he finally believed me when I told him we would have to find alternative living arrangements until we could file an insurance claim and try to recover. He was at a loss for words and became so distraught that he left work early to see the severity of the damage for himself. I waited for him, and we cried in each other's arms. Everything was gone. Clothing, appliances, important documents, and all the keepsakes, mementos, and pictures we had accumulated throughout the years. None of these things could ever be replaced. We were left with our memories and our son.

We were now homeless. I had friends I could count on to house me and my son. My husband reached out to his family, who allowed him to stay with them. Our family was split up. There were many questions to be answered, but that was best left to the authorities.

One humanitarian decision intended to help an abused woman and her child cost me my home and everything inside it. But it could have cost me a lot more. An act of kindness had become the catalyst of a domino effect leading to an unimaginable situation. There was approximately $50,000 to $60,000 worth of damage, and insurance refused to cover it because the damage was determined to be caused by arson.

I got very little sleep that night. The next morning, I called the hospital where I worked to explain what happened and that I would need at least a few hours to purchase a new uniform. The person I was speaking to asked if it was a sick call.

In a tone she probably did not deserve, I roared, "No, I do not know what kind of reason you can use! I just cannot come in until I buy a uniform! I have no work clothes!"

Later in the day, I explained to my supervisor the details of the situation and that I had nothing left to wear. I enjoyed a good relationship with my bosses and colleagues. When I was able to report to work at the hospital, the staff had raised money for me to buy new uniforms. The Red Cross also got involved and donated things to help us get back on our feet.

I was very grateful for these gestures, but with no help from the insurance company, I needed money and a whole lot of it. There would be no vacations this year or the next and perhaps the one after that. It was time to work and raise money.

I felt guilty because my decision to move in with a friend in need had destabilized the lives of many people. Not only were the lives of my husband and my son unbalanced, but so were the lives of the people who stepped in to lend a hand.

Research: Homelessness

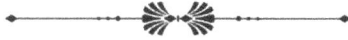

I have reason to believe that Kettlyne never imagined that one day she would experience homelessness. Why should she? Kettlyne had a home that she was willing to share with her friends and loved ones when needed. This just demonstrates the fragility of our security networks. When people think of homelessness, they generally conceive it as a third-world problem where poverty is pervasive. Still, in reality, it is a plight in almost every country, even in an industrialized civilization such as America. Homelessness is an ever-increasing problem, with no real improvements in the policies. Most homeless people in the United States seek refuge in crowded shelters, sustained by private donations with barely any funds from the government.

Definition of Homelessness

Homelessness is defined by many people in many complicated ways, but let us take this simple definition. According to David Hulchanski, it is about inadequate housing, inadequate income, and a lack of appropriate social support.

According to *The Homeless Hub,* homelessness is an intense form of poverty characterized by inconsistent or unstable housing and a lack of adequate income, healthcare resources, and social support. This definition includes people who are conclusively homeless (those living on the streets), shelter dwellers (people staying temporarily in emergency shelters or hostels), the "hidden homeless" (people staying temporarily with friends or family), and others who technically have a place to live but are "at-risk" of homelessness.

Gender and Individual Homelessness

The way homelessness is measured is generally a "point-in-time" count of people sleeping either on the streets or in shelters. Basically, this data reflects the number of homeless people on a given night. Housing and Urban Development is an important source of information. It releases the Annual Homeless Assessment Report to Congress (AHARC) by calculating "point-in-time" homelessness in late January of each year. The data on "Continuums of Care" (COC) come from active counts that are taken at the community level by walking around the streets, using long-established methodologies.

Men and Women

A formidable majority of men are counted every year in the point-in-time count to be homeless. Men are also more likely to be unsheltered than women. During the 2018 point-in-time (PiT) count, 67% of the homeless were men. According to the demographics, there are 260,284 homeless men and 106,119 homeless women. Hence there are nearly 70% men comprising the majority of individuals experiencing homelessness, and 29% women. The final percent includes transgender and non-binary individuals.

At a more local level, the data shows that 97% of men are covering the most individuals experiencing homelessness in almost all CoCs. When it comes to unsheltered homelessness, it has been on the rise for almost the last two years now. There is only a slight difference between the percentage of men and women among unsheltered homelessness, men comprising 49% and women 45%.

Nationally in the United States' general population, 21.5 men and 8.3 women experience homelessness per 10,000 people. The highest per capita rate of homeless individuals is in Washington, D.C., with men being 104.6 and women being 34.4, almost double the rate in California at 52.5 and 19.9 for men and women, respectively.

During HUD's Annual Point-in-Time Count in January 2019, seventeen out of every 10,000 people in the United States were experiencing homelessness on one night. These 567,715 people represent a cross-section of America, belonging to every region of the country, gender category, family status, and racial/ethnic group.

Children

Each year in America, a startling number of 2.5 million children experience homelessness. This notably high number represents one in every thirty children in the United States. In 2016, almost 1.3 million children under six years old experienced homelessness. On a single night in January 2018, 111,592 children were experiencing homelessness. Thirty-three percent of people enduring homelessness lived in families with children. More than half of all homeless families with children lived in just four states: California, Florida, Massachusetts, and New York.

During the 2016-2017 school years, nearly 1.4 million children enrolled in public schools experienced homelessness. Additionally, a report by Voices of Youth Count from the University of Chicago reported 4.2 million teens and young adults suffer homelessness yearly.

Homelessness and Mental Health

It is unbelievable that the United States, the twelfth richest country globally, can have such a staggering amount of homelessness at half a million people on any given night. There are numerous reasons behind this plague, including domestic abuse, home displacement, substance abuse, and family rejection, leading to higher rates of depression, substance misuse or addiction, and/or diagnosed or undiagnosed mental illness, and suicidal thoughts. As seen in Kettlyne's case, at times, these causes may even involve adjacent families. It was her friend who was experiencing domestic abuse, but Kettlyne's home situation was affected all the same simply because she knew the victim and was offering assistance.

The relation between homelessness and mental health is two-way, as many researchers accept. Poor mental health may cause behavioral and cognitive problems, leading to difficulties in normal functioning such as maintaining a job or a stable income, followed by homelessness. On the other hand, studies have shown that homelessness exacerbates mental illness. This is because the experience of being homeless is extremely traumatic. The person is exposed to dangers and threats that can cause acute stress and make a person more prone to many mental illnesses.

The most common disorders found among the homeless are affective disorders such as depression, anxiety, bipolar, substance abuse, and schizophrenia. Homelessness while enduring a mental illness makes survival even more arduous. Studies reveal that homeless mentally challenged people have more encounters with the criminal justice system than those not homeless. They have more psychotic interactions with police and are more likely to be victimized.

Mothers are found to be at a greater risk. Researchers have found that mothers who experience postpartum depression are more likely to suffer homelessness in the years to come. A significant study on children and homelessness tracking 17,000 children in Denmark revealed a higher prevalence of psychiatric disorders, including substance abuse, among adolescents with a mother or both parents with a history of homelessness.

Research has also shown the drastic effects of homelessness on child development and how it jeopardizes their future. Homeless children face serious risks. It threatens their ability to succeed and their future well-being. Health problems, hunger, poor nutrition, anxiety, depression, behavioral problems, educational underachievement, and developmental delays are serious concerns. Another study on the influence of housing instability on anxiety, locus of control (LOC), behavior, and academic performance reinforced that children who experienced more incidents of homelessness had more significant problems with behavior and anxiety. Their GPA is not affected initially by the housing issues but by the locus of control, behavioral issues, and anxiety caused by housing variables.

How to Provide Support?

There is without a doubt much that needs to be done. Many private services are trying their best to provide support for the homeless, including services that provide the homeless individuals and families with temporary and permanent housing services and assist them until they can stand on their own feet. This is the most appropriate way of providing support, as many studies show that homeless people suffering from mental health issues have improved significantly when provided with stable housing. In addition, the children need to get appropriate support to be made independent and become capable of supporting themselves in the future. According to *Ballin,* "Shelters need to have the supportive services to help homeless youth eventually transition to independent living in the community, services need to include education, employment, health, and mental health."

However, although many private services are working hard to eliminate homelessness, they simply do not have the resources to cope with the situation. Therefore, the government needs to exert the most responsibility. Throughout the United States, there are only 11,364 community housing and homeless shelters. They either do not offer or are not capable of offering all of the support that homeless individuals need. Without sufficient support and funding from the government, the system can not keep up because the number of homeless individuals and families is far larger than private services can handle. Of course, every individual can provide support on his/her own level and according to their capacity, but the truth is that the problem is too systematic to be solved this way.

Conclusion

Homelessness is not a national problem. Instead, it is a global one. It is not caused by laziness or the personal inability of a person to earn money. Instead, it can be caused by an economic crisis, mental health conditions, displacement from family, loss of home due to natural disasters, etc. Kettlyne had a home and two jobs, but this was not enough to protect her from an unfortunate incident. She did not have the financial resources to cope adequately with the setback, which is not unusual even for gainfully employed medical professionals. This is not the time to shame people who are experiencing such traumatic events. Instead, it is a time to step forward and provide any help and support that can put even a single person out of misery. And it is a time to raise a voice against the system so this can end for good.

Chapter 2
Happy, Not-So-Happy Birthday

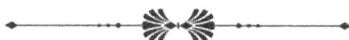

———— ⁂ ————

With everything that was going on in my life, the last thing on my mind was my birthday. A couple of days after the destructive fire, I was heading to work for a little overtime. It was an effective way to deal with the new normal I was experiencing. No longer able to enjoy the luxury and independence of my own home, I was sleeping at a friend's house, a temporary haven that could accommodate my baby and me. Although I was grateful for the help, it was not comfortable. On top of that, a surprise houseguest can quickly overstay their welcome. I had to resolve my personal problems and move out before I became a burden.

My twenty-fourth birthday was on Saturday, December 22, 2001. That morning, I was supposed to be on my day off. Instead of enjoying the time with my family, I volunteered to work. Hospitals are notoriously short-staffed, and getting extra work is just a matter of speaking up. I needed all the hours I could get for the extra cash. Work not only took my mind off my problems but also helped me suppress feelings of guilt. I felt responsible, and working twice as much to make up for the damage allowed for consolatory peace of mind. Therefore, any shift that anyone wanted to surrender to me was much appreciated. And any time the hospital was short-staffed, I could be counted on to fill the spot.

It was about six in the morning and still dark, with sunrise approaching fast. As I dropped off my son at the babysitter's house, I realized I had forgotten my cellphone at my temporary home. It was too late to backtrack. I had to punch a time clock soon. Within minutes I jumped onto Interstate 95 southbound and began the usual ten-mile trek to work. As a matter of habit, I tried to casually ease into the inside lane seeking safety from drivers entering the freeway.

In the rearview mirror, I noticed a vehicle on my right coming up fast and swerving. I thought, "I better let this car pass by before he ends up doing something really crazy." I lightly pressed the brake and took frequent glances to make sure I was not in danger. Other cars were their best to steer clear of the erratic vehicle that looked like it was about to lose control. It was beyond carelessness. It was beyond mere fatigue. There was no doubt in my mind the driver was impaired.

As the vehicle closed the distance between us, it appeared it would pass on the far outside lane with room to spare. I continued to slow down and took my eyes off the mirror to glance right and confirm the scare was over as the car rolled by. However, instead of seeing what I was expecting, headlights were coming directly toward me. The oncoming vehicle had whipped across the freeway, crossing four lanes of traffic.

Time slowed to a crawl as so many things went through my mind. One thought was, "I hope he does not hit my car." Another was, "More insurance issues." And then I thought about my son just before a side impact so forceful that it slammed my car into the median barrier and flipped it completely upside down. The whirling motion and jarring halt were so disorienting that I was unaware the impact had collapsed the engine onto my legs. As I recovered from the shock, the vehicle that hit me immediately fled the scene of the accident. For all intents and purposes, the driver left me for dead.

Somehow, I had not lost consciousness. I do not recall the airbags deploying in my 1999 Toyota Previa, but I am sure they had a lot to do with me not sustaining head injuries. I can also attest that the minivan had a very, very good seatbelt that prevented me from being ejected onto the asphalt or oncoming traffic. Wedged in tight and strapped in place upside-down, a wave of panic began to form in the center of my chest. "No!" I said aloud and took a deep breath, forcing myself to calm down. Then, I realized there was no cellphone within reach to call for help.

Over the sounds of hissing and creaking, I could hear traffic. It was still dark, and vehicles with curious drivers slowed but continued about their business. In the present day, there are public service patrols and traffic cameras that monitor hazardous road conditions and detrimental incidents. At the beginning of the new millennium, however, technology and the city's budget did not allow for either convenience. I was sure the passersby would call 9-1-1. Help would arrive, but in ten minutes, fifteen minutes…when?

There was nothing I could do but wait and listen for someone to stop. Agonizing seconds turned into minutes. It felt like I had been trapped in that vehicle for an eternity. Whenever I tried to free myself, all I succeeded in doing was sliding my torso closer to the dashboard and tightening the snugness of the seatbelt. I stopped resisting the pull of gravity and let my arms fall over my head so that I could push myself up. Unfortunately, it did not work, and the sensation of being suffocated and strangled at the same time was terrifying. To make matters worse, the pungent fumes from the fuel, oil, and battery acid were making it hard to breathe.

As the light of dawn pushed back the gloom, it helped to distract me from the discomfort. I tried to get my bearings and find my purse. I considered tossing it out onto the road to attract attention. It was then I began to feel a burning sensation in both my legs. To say it frightened me is an understatement. I looked for flames and cautiously reached toward the warmth only to draw back in fear. I did not want to burn, but there was no fire. Instead, what I had felt was blood trickling down and painting the white uniform that I had worn perhaps once before a distinct red color. For a fleeting second, I was comforted by the thought that I would painlessly bleed out before flames or an explosion killed me.

The world began to push in on me. I looked into the rearview mirror awaiting release from the troubles and hardships of daily life. Staring back at me was the mother of a young child, a little boy who would one day wonder what went wrong on December 22, 2001, the day his mother was supposed to have celebrated her twenty-fourth birthday. He would question if anything could have been done to prevent what happened to his mom on that fateful day.

The thought of my son possibly growing up without a mother gave me the strength to attempt to get myself out, but I did not know-how. It was then a vehicle stopped. A woman whose face I could not see crouched next to me and introduced herself. I do not recall her name. I reached out, took her outstretched hand, and begged her to free me before the car exploded. She assured me there was no fire and urged me not to move until help arrived. It was difficult to be still with the seatbelt cutting into my neck.

Finally, the woman took notice and cut the strap with trauma shears. I recognized the handy tool used by healthcare professionals and asked where she worked. As it turned out, we had the same employer, and she was also on her way to work. If I am not mistaken, the angel of mercy who comforted me was a pediatric physician. I told her I worked in the emergency department as an EMT technician. She instructed me not to move as we spoke. Once the lights and sirens arrived, the woman moved away to allow the paramedics to do their work.

Knowing how hard the men and women from fire rescue work, I answered every question they asked with an apology. One of them shimmied into my car on his back with a flashlight to get a better look at my legs. The paramedic asked if I was having trouble breathing, and I told him I was better after the doctor cut the seatbelt. My response baffled the rescuers. One of them stated he did not see anyone at the scene when they arrived. They assumed that I was hallucinating even though I pointed out that my seatbelt had to be cut by someone because I couldn't do it on my own. I continued to ramble on as they tried to stop the bleeding. At one point, I told the paramedics that my son was in the back seat and sent them into a panic. Thankfully, my son was not in the car, and the paramedics continued to rescue me from the car. The burning sensation on my legs, the blood loss, and the shock were taking their toll on me.

There was a distressed look in the faces of my rescuers as they struggled to lift and hold the floorboard in a position in which I could be extricated. With both of my legs pinned under the dashboard and compressed by the brake and accelerator pedals, the problem was far from over. I give them credit for moving quickly. The tools used to free me were canvass straps and blocks of wood. The release endeavor tore up my feet and may have worsened the lower extremity injuries I had sustained. However, I could not complain. I was alive and grateful for the efforts of these heroes, dedicated professionals who risk their lives on a daily basis. I was happy to be out of the wreckage. I wanted to see my son again.

Within seconds of being pulled out of the vehicle, I was placed on a backboard, a cervical collar was applied, and I was carried onto a helicopter. The last thing I remember was a lot of noise and feeling very cold before losing consciousness. At the time, I did not know the extent of my injuries. I had bilateral tibia fibula fractures and crush injuries from the knees down. Both legs were severely damaged.

When I awoke hours later, I was in the recovery area of a trauma emergency department. Given that I was transported in a helicopter, I knew exactly where I was. This was the county hospital where I worked. There were monitors and gizmos all around me, but I fixed my gaze on a lonely clock hanging on a wall at the far end of the room. It was lunchtime, but I wondered if it was the same day or if I had slept through the morning and into the next day.

The next thing to capture my attention were three pink balloons tied to a pole holding an IV pump. The sight was quite perplexing until I heard a familiar voice wish me a happy birthday. I gingerly turned my head to meet the gaze of my closest friend, Sally. We had been like sisters since the seventh grade. The rush of joy brought a big smile to my face.

I should not have been surprised to see her at my side. Sally was a fellow hospital employee, a nurse with a few years of experience. When I was hired, I had listed her as my next of kin. Sally was the only contact person in my medical file. She had barely begun her shift when word of my situation reached her. The employees on her floor took over her job duties, and an administrator escorted her to where I was.

"Do you want me to sing to you?" Sally asked, tugging at the balloons.

I shook my head and whispered, "No…glad you remembered."

She looked away and proclaimed, "Well, that's okay. It has not really been a day deserving of celebration."

Her tone made me suspicious. I drew an audible breath that got Sally's attention and uttered an unrestrained groan in an attempt to clear my throat. There were so many questions, but my mouth was so dry. I motioned for a sip of water, but Sally advised me I could not have a drink as tears welled up in her eyes.

"Please tell me what is wrong?" I implored.

"I'm sorry," she appealed. "I didn't mean to frighten you."

Sally quickly explained the extent of the injuries to me, her voice cracking with emotion. The date was still December 22. Only a handful of hours, a short time, had passed since I was involved in the accident. It was bad. And this woman at my side – my friend, my confidant, my sister – was sharing every ounce of my suffering. Her face smeared with tears, she paused to look for paper towels to dry her face.

The new knowledge was overwhelming. I had not released a single tear. Could someone be too distressed to cry? I certainly felt that way.

When Sally arrived at the trauma department, while she was not allowed access to the treatment area, she acted as an advocate on my behalf. She knew my allergies. She knew my medical conditions. Sally was the most qualified candidate for this role. My mother and my husband could not be the gatekeepers of my healthcare. Undoubtedly, the trauma team assumed Sally was my sister or another immediate family member. And I am very grateful it played out in this way because Sally spoke up when the medical residents expressed that they were planning to perform a double amputation of my lower extremities. She put a halt to the pending surgical intervention by adamantly telling them that living without legs would not happen. Sally requested to speak to the chief of orthopedics and asked him to explore other treatment options, something better than bilateral lower extremity amputation.

Before long, the eagerly awaited physician appeared. He was a tall man with a perpetual frown that undoubtedly unsettled most patients under his care. He explained that he had examined the diagnostic imaging results, and, despite the extensive damage, he was willing to do his best to save my legs. With a shrug, he estimated that it would take approximately seven operations and that it would be a long and difficult road to recovery.

The man had the bedside manner of a lumberjack, but his no-nonsense approach was quite refreshing. I was thrilled that he would try to repair my legs and thanked him profusely. Sally stepped in and redirected the conversation back to the multiple surgeries. As they spoke, the doctor slipped on a pair of gloves and pulled at the bandages around my feet to palpate the pulses of my damaged extremities. His touch burned as if he had pressed hot coals to my skin. I instinctively pulled away and regretted it.

My legs were still very much injured, only immobilized to prevent further damage and promote circulation. I had been stabilized for surgery with large-bore intravenous access ports on each arm, an indwelling urinary catheter, and other bells and whistles. There was no pain as long as I did not move. However, even a deep breath was excruciating.

Sally noticed my intense discomfort and asked the physician to stop. He gingerly withdrew his hands and asked if Sally was my healthcare proxy.

"Yes!" I answered. Absolutely and emphatically, "Yes."

Once I was administered pain medication, I could not make informed decisions. No amount of explanation would provide them a comprehensive understanding of the significance of a surgical procedure. Sally had shown her grit, and I needed to empower her with decision-making authority. Bring on the paperwork!

The doctor explained the new intervention to both of us, answered a few questions, and stated that he would return soon with a surgical consent form. Then, he spun on his heels and walked away, declaring that he would order pain medication. When he departed, he took the heaviness in the room with him. Sally and I celebrated the victory and the not-so-happy birthday.

I asked if she had spoken to my mother or my husband. Sally did not have their contact numbers. Since both of my loved ones were at work, there was no need to break the news to them just yet. I figured it would be best to wait until quitting time so that my husband could pick up my mother and bring her for a quick visit. The babysitter would have to step up and care for my son until my mother, and I determined what we would do.

For the rest of the day, I went in and out of a blissful stupor whenever nurses administered medication. I was awake when my mother and husband arrived. They took it better than I had imagined. Well, at least my mother did. My husband bowed his head in silence for a long moment before walking out of the room. Sally drove my mother to the babysitter's home to pick up my son.

Seven operations! Seven invasive procedures. It was all I could think about.

Every morning the trauma team paid me a visit, including, but not limited to, the chief of orthopedics and his residents. During their pre-dawn rounds, it sometimes felt as if they forgot that I was a patient and treated me like an object by indelicately pulling off bandages to assess the wounds. Given that it was morning shift change, despite my pleas to the nursing staff, I was not always pre-medicated before the heavy-handed inspection and palpation began. I must admit, I got tired of routinely waking up to insurmountable pain. I understood the team had to perform their rounds in an expeditious manner in order to communicate the plan of care to one another and get to the hands-on work as soon as possible. Still, the fact that they were in my presence talking about me as if I was not conscious was irritating. Had they known I was a fellow medical professional and not naïve to the medical jargon, perhaps they would have been more thoughtful. I eventually confronted the team and asked to be involved in the discussion, but, more importantly, I asked to be medicated before being examined.

After every surgical procedure, there was rehabilitation. It was the same routine every time, and it seemed endless, always difficult, always painful. Whenever a little progress was made, it was time for another surgical procedure. I felt defeated due to constant, severe pain. If it is at all possible, expecting the pain was worse than experiencing it. It was also emotionally debilitating knowing that if the sequence of surgeries and rehabilitation did not go well, there was the likelihood I would never walk again.

By surgery number four, I began to tire of the endless and cumbersome therapy. Imagine running a race, and every fifty paces, officials sent you back to the starting line. You could see the finish line in the distance, but it seemed impossible to reach it. I kept putting myself through a daily, constant struggle to get better, only to end up starting all over again. I wondered if it was worth the effort. It seemed that all aspects of the cure to my affliction were working against me.

For example, there were steroid injections that led to weight gain that resulted in greater difficulty getting out of bed. The pain medication sometimes worked for background pain but not for sudden piercing pain spikes that accompany physical therapy exercises. Also, being a patient in the healthcare institution where I worked and took pride in helping the needy had become unpleasant. I felt as if my old colleagues were watching my decline and judging me.

I did not want to be dependent on anyone. I did not want anyone looking at me. Yes, it sounds like I had metamorphosized into a moody diva, but helplessness is a harsh reality. I slipped into woeful depression, or perhaps it could be better described as a distressing disappointment. In frustration, I would cry myself to sleep every night and wake up crying every morning. Would I have been better off as an amputee? At least the surgeries and the accompanying pain would have stopped.

I was too deep into my funk to recognize that the staff, my colleagues and friends, were paying more attention to me than they were to other patients. Instead of feeling like a charity case, I should have felt honored that everyone was putting extra effort into helping me. It was not until Emmanuel, a friend who worked in the emergency department, began to drop by that I was able to get motivated once more.

When I began my employment, Emmanuel was my preceptor. He had just returned to work after recuperating from a traumatic automobile accident in which he sustained multiple injuries to the extent in which he required facial reconstruction surgery. Emmanuel was in the same position I was now in, if not much worse. When I met him, his wounds were completely healed but quite visible.

One evening after his shift, when he visited me for the first time, he grinned from ear to ear like the fictional Cheshire Cat and asked, "Do you know how lucky you are?" With the index finger of his right hand, he traced the scar that ran across his left eyelid, the bridge of his nose, and down his right cheek.

Emmanuel knew what I was going through more than most people and tried to put it into perspective for me. His message was simple to grasp. He was there to communicate that the injuries could have been worse, more aesthetically noticeable, more debilitating, crippling, and even fatal.

He asked if I was interested in going for a ride, and even though I declined, even though I did not want to be bothered, I soon found myself in a wheelchair being paraded through endless hallways I had never visited before. It was inevitable running into patients, young and old, who were suffering from chronic and acute conditions that eclipsed my injuries.

"Look at that poor man," Emmanuel would point out. "Do not stare! You are so rude!"

Before the experience got old, we ended up at the top of the tallest parking garage. On the southeast corner of the structure, although the ocean remained out of sight, the cruise ships at the Port of Miami could be seen. Emmanuel told me that he came up here as often as he could because the view reminded him of his home in the Philippines.

As the sun went down in the west, in an earnest tone, Emmanuel asked if I had seen the man with four arms and two heads.

"No," I respond with a laugh, "but I know where you are going with this."

"Good," he rejoiced in a slow and wobbly voice. "Then I won't have to point out the man with no legs?"

I tried my best to hold a grimace and keep from laughing at his silliness, but we exchanged a glance that broke me down. I smiled. I laughed.

"I needed this," I confided. "I needed to laugh because I do not want to cry anymore."

Emmanuel visited routinely. He looked out for me and understood my situation because he could relate to what I was feeling. Through tales of his journey toward a full recovery, through the courage in his eyes, I found strength.

"Giving up is believing in weakness," he would often say.

Slowly but surely, Emmanuel got me back into the physical therapy exercise regimen. He encouraged me to interact with other patients who were going through similar situations to relate and connect. I began to look at the arduous rehab exercises through a different lens. A lot of patients were going through the same difficulties I was experiencing. Some faltered, some quit, and others persevered. I soon found myself helping people who were struggling on the road to recovery. I must admit, you learn a lot about your own frailties when you make the effort to help others.

A visit from my son also proved to have a beneficial effect on my level of motivation.

Throughout my time in the hospital, my mother would routinely bring my son for visits. At the tender age of three, he was not allowed into the area where I was staying, but I could meet them outside. As joyful as these reunions were, they were hard on him. He could not understand why Mommy could not come home. I tried my best to explain that I was hurt and needed to get better.

It was not hard keeping him from seeing the stabilization bars and metal rings encircling my legs. However, one day the sheet that I guardedly kept tucked tight lifted just enough for my son to catch a glimpse of the orthopedic hardware. He was horrified. My little boy clutched his hands to his chest and began to cry.

In the calmest tone I could muster, I tried to paint the simplest possible terms that a toddler would easily understand that Mommy was almost better. It took a while for the sobbing to subside, but he was not about to let it go. Finally, my baby took it upon himself to instruct me on how to fix my legs. I watched him innocently describe the process I should follow to get up, stretch, and exercise my legs. He even went as far as demonstrating how to position my lower extremities to get out of the wheelchair without falling.

"You can do it," he assured me.

My son was so determined to try everything within his power to help his mother recover. His enthusiasm for me to get better gave me an extra boost of motivation to continue getting the help I needed. Suddenly, the journey was not just about me. It was about us. My baby needed me.

Research: Depression

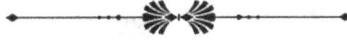

As Kettlyne was lying on the hospital bed, depression started to sink in. To be so young and vibrant in one moment and then suddenly losing independence and autonomy due to a terrible event such as this is not easy to accept.

Depression, formally known as clinical depression or Major Depressive Disorder, is a serious medical condition. It is a form of depressive disorder that causes severe symptoms affecting the way a person thinks, feels, and behaves. The symptoms generally include depressed mood, loss of interest, hopelessness, sleep and appetite disturbances, and/or suicidal ideation or attempts.

For many years now, the word "depression" has been used offhandedly to the point of losing the gravity of what it actually represents. To be more precise, it is more than just a bad or a sad day or minor inconvenience. It is not just a "mood." To be diagnosed with depression, proper scientific testing and diagnostic evaluations are required by a professional. And similarly, proper treatment is required for its treatment.

Types of Depression

According to the Diagnostic and Statistical Manual of Mental Disorders, Fifth Edition (DSM-5), Depressive disorders include major depressive disorder, mood dysregulation disorder, persistent depressive disorder (dysthymia), premenstrual dysphoric disorder, substance/medication-induced depressive disorder, and depressive disorder due to another medical condition. In addition, there are other types of depression such as Bipolar Disorder—known as "manic depression"—seasonal affective disorder (SAD), and postpartum depression.

Though the triggers and contexts of depression vary, they share common features such as sadness, a feeling of emptiness, or irritable mood, accompanied by somatic and cognitive changes that significantly affect the individual's capacity to function. The variables found in depression are duration, timing, or presumed cause. For example, the diagnosis for major depressive disorder requires the symptoms to be present for at least two weeks.

Invisible Depression

Sometimes depression is hard to detect, not only in others but also in oneself. We need to realize that while most people are good at projecting a sense of normalcy and may seem "happy," not everyone is in tune with their inner world, and not everyone is good at introspection. Many people find it hard to know and accept their emotions and thoughts, while many stay completely oblivious.

On the other hand, some people know exactly what they feel and actively try to hide it from others. There are many terms given to this phenomenon. Some call it invisible or "concealed" depression. Others refer to it as *Smiling Depression,* indicating that a person can be in the pits of depression and still be smiling in front of the world, hiding everything they are going through. For people suffering from depression, smiling is a kind of defense mechanism, a façade of being "well."

Why Do People Hide Their Depression?

There are many reasons people put on this persona, the first and most prominent being the stigma around mental health. For example, it is generally more difficult for men to reach out as they fear being perceived as weak. The typical response to setbacks is to "man up." Other than the stigmas, some people find it hard to share personal feelings. They worry about worrying others, and the guilt of being "weak" masks their distress. With social media portraying everything and everyone as perfectly happy, a common perception of unrealistic happiness results. People suffering from depression and other mental health conditions think that they are the only ones with unhappy feelings, and everyone else is just happy, which is far from reality. This false image stops them from reaching out for help. In reality, people suffering from depression are not the only ones, and social media is not a true reflection of reality.

How to Identify Depression

If we learn about the symptoms and signs of depression, we can identify them in ourselves and others. Everyone gets sad every now and then, so how can we separate normal mood changes from depression? The first thing to notice is a loss of interest in the things and activities that a person usually finds interesting. The next thing is to look for disturbances in eating and sleeping. In depression, these two will either get abnormally low or high. Examples would be if a person starts eating more portions than they usually do (binge eating) or starts eating significantly less, or if a person starts sleeping a lot (hypersomnia) or loses sleep (insomnia). At this point, we can notice the irritability in mood and overwhelming emotions.

Most importantly, we can look for warning signs, particularly suicide, and talk about it if we suspect anything or talk to others if such thoughts occur. In concealed depression, the risk of suicide is higher, as generally depressed people find it hard to get up, and due to loss of energy, they can barely plan for suicide. But in smiling depression, a person usually occupies themselves with an excess of work or destructive habits (like drinking or smoking) to hide their depression, so they have more energy to attempt suicide.

When to Seek Help?

Watch for symptoms of depression (weight loss, feelings of "emptiness" and sadness, increasing disinterest in hobbies and activities a person usually enjoys, sleep disturbance, loss of energy, increased irritability, lowered self-esteem, trouble concentrating, and contemplating suicide). Suppose a person has five or more of the symptoms listed above for more than two weeks nearly every day. In that case, it is time to consult with a professional, especially if these symptoms interfere with daily life and normal functioning.

Though there is no simple checklist to follow if a person feels like they cannot handle their emotional or mental state and needs to reach out for help at any given moment, depressed individuals may confide in their close friends or loved ones. This is a good approach. However, you may feel like it is not enough. After all, they are not professionals. They can only listen and not provide proper treatment. It is then that we know it is time to reach out for professional help.

How to Seek Help

Seeking help for your mental health can be difficult, but once you take the first step, you will realize that it is not as horrible as it is usually portrayed. A person can ask and confide in family and friends first to let them know that they need professional help. The support from loved ones is helpful to go forward. They can help find a suitable mental health professional and even accompany them to the first few appointments.

In Kettlyne's case, a friend helped identify her situation and worked to help get her on a path to recovery. But if someone does not feel comfortable talking about their mental health with family or friends, it is entirely okay to reach for professional help directly. You can get professional help and treatment from a clinical psychologist, psychiatrist, social worker, or a licensed mental health counselor. Mental health services can also be reached through your local hospital, community mental health centers, university, or medical school-affiliated mental health clinics.

Why is it Important to Seek Help?

The importance of seeking professional help for depression lies in the simple fact that it improves your quality of life. Depression affects normal life functioning, and getting treatment means that you are availing a basic necessity of good and better health. In Kettlyne's case, her depression prevented her from taking full advantage of the physical rehabilitation she needed to recover from the surgeries. Living with depression or any mental health illness and not getting treatment means risking adverse effects on your life. British Medical Journal published a study in 2012 revealing that even mild mental health problems can lead to a lower life expectancy.

It is crucial to acknowledge that depression does unfold itself not only mentally but also physically. The person also has to deal with somatic symptoms and emotions. Thus, treatment is better for mental health and physical health. In addition, research has indicated that mental health issues weaken the immune system. Therefore, by not seeking professional help, many health factors are damaged. There are many forms of treatment a person can choose, from therapy to medication, but the important thing is to take a step toward a healthier life.

Prevalence of Depression

Tens of millions of people are affected by mental health issues in the United States, and Depression is the most prevalent, representing 99% of all mind-brain illnesses (Schizophrenia and major psychotic illness represent the remaining 1%). In the United States, depression affects over 18 million people in any given year and is the prime agent of disability for ages 15-44 years. According to the Centers for Disease Control and Prevention (CDC), every 12 minutes, a person commits suicide in the U.S. Major depression is regarded as a significant cause of suicide.

Among Adults

According to the data collected in 2017 in the National Survey on Drug Use and Health Methodological Summary and Definitions, at least 17.3 million adults in the United States were verified to have had at least one major depressive episode. This number represented 7.1% of all U.S. adults. Female adults showed a higher percentage (8.7%) than male adults (5.3%). The episodes were more significant for the age group 18-25. An estimated 1 million U.S. adults aged 18 or older experienced at least one major depressive episode with severe impairment. This staggering number of cases represents 4.5% of all U.S. adults.

Among Adolescents

According to the 2017 National Survey on Drug Use and Health (NSDUH) conducted by the National Institute of Mental Health (NIMH), 3.2 million adolescents aged 12 to 17 in the United States have experienced at least one major depressive episode, representing 13.3% of the U.S. adolescent population. It is significantly higher among adolescent females (20.0%) compared to males (6.8%). There are also 3 million adolescents aged 12 to 17 in the United States who had at least one major depressive episode with severe impairment, representing 9.4% of the U.S. adolescent population.

In the United States, depression kills over 41,000 people a year. In comparison, homicide claims less than 16,000 lives each year, according to 2013 CDC statistics. Globally, 300 million people are affected by depression, regardless of culture, age, gender, religion, race, or economic status.

Research: Post Traumatic Stress Syndrome

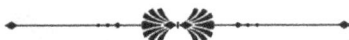

Post-Traumatic Stress Disorder (PTSD) is a chronic impairment disorder that triggers a spectrum of psycho-emotional and physio-pathological consequences in individuals who experienced or witnessed a traumatic event (Miao et al., 2018). The distressing situations are life-threatening and could be a natural catastrophe, accident, combat exposure, sexual assault, financial problem, or anything threatening you with death. Kettlyne experienced two incidents that would certainly be events that could lead to PTSD-either the house fire or the car accident.

According to the findings of Dahlby & Kerr (2020), 1 out of 11 people is diagnosed with PTSD in their lifetime, affecting approximately 3.5% of the U.S. population annually regardless of ethnicity, nationality, culture, or age. In 1990, around 5.2 million American adults aged 18 to 54 suffered from this anxiety disorder, costing an estimated 46.6 billion dollars for treatment (Choi et al., 2021). Untreated PTSD adversely affects day-to-day functioning, relationships, physical health, and the ability to enjoy life. Over 80% of individuals with long-standing PTSD develop a higher risk for mental health problems like depression, anxiety, rebellious behavior, and Attention Deficit Hyperactivity Disorder (Sangalang et al., 2018). Also, it may influence people to engage in riskier and health-compromising behaviors, such as alcohol or other substance abuse. These factors combine to put a great strain on a person's body and increase the hazard for physical health problems and illness. This research aims to analyze the effect of PTSD on mental health in women, men, and children supported by statistics.

Discussion

PTSD results in severe stress and damaging consequences for survivors and their families. Although the majority of the individuals cope with the trauma over time, many survivors experience long-lasting problems, both chronic and severe.

The complications may include:

- Anxiety
- Indignity
- Aggression
- Nightmares
- Terror
- Insomnia
- Somatic disturbances
- Loss of trust
- Social isolation
- Difficulty with intimate relationships
- Suicidal behaviors

The studies reveal that working women and those who belong to underprivileged populations are at greater risk for experiencing undesirable consequences following traumatic events such as sexual abuse and harassment. They exhibit more sensitivity to stimuli that remind them of the trauma and may experience physical symptoms, including headaches, gastrointestinal problems, and sexual dysfunction. In addition, the survivor women often wait for years to seek help while others never receive any treatment due to shame, whether it is a personal shame or the fear of being shamed by others.

Many children and teenagers with PTSD experience similar problems to adults, like suicidal thoughts and substance abuse. They express their distress in different ways. For example, some of them re-live the incident in flashback episodes, especially when exposed to particular situations or objects. Some lose interest in performing daily activities, become socially withdrawn, or exhibit extreme temper tantrums. Many older children have terrifying dreams with ambiguous content rather than dreams repeating the traumatic event.

According to the National Vietnam Veterans Readjustment studies, 75% of male Vietnam veterans who had PTSD were also diagnosed with alcohol abuse, 44% had a diagnosis of generalized anxiety disorder, and about 20% were diagnosed with dysthymia depression throughout their lives. In addition, they were also at increased risk for trauma such as deadly motor vehicle accidents and suicide (Steenkamp et al., 2017). Whereas 44% of female Vietnam veterans who had PTSD had a lifetime diagnosis of depression (Steenkamp et al., 2017).

Prevalence of PTSD and Statistics

PTSD is emerging as a major health problem in America. The National Center for PTSD estimates approximately 3.6% of adults developed PTSD in the past year (Dauphin, 2020). Six out of ten men and five out of ten working women experience at least one trauma in their lives, and an estimated 1.8% of men and 5.2% of adult women develop PTSD symptoms (Dauphin, 2020). The figures indicate that PTSD is more common in women than in men. However, men seem to experience more traumatic events during their lifetime than women. Whereas about 15 – 43% of girls and 14 – 43% of boys go through at least one drastic event from which 3 – 15% of girls and 1– 6% of boys develop PTSD (Foa et al., 2017).

Women are more likely to experience sexual assault and childhood physical abuse, whereas men are more likely to experience accidents, physical assault, or instances of violence and death. PTSD in children is associated with harsh parenting styles, bad accidents, physical or emotional abuse, violent personal attacks, or invasive medical trials, particularly for children younger than age 6. It can lead to detrimental effects on their mental health, such as difficulty in school and the development of phobias.

Symptoms of PTSD

The symptoms of PTSD are commonly divided into four types:

- Intrusive memories
- Avoidance
- Negative changes in thinking, feelings, and temperament
- Variations in physical and emotional reactions

Symptoms vary from person to person with the progression of time. They may begin within a month of a traumatic event or may not appear until years after the event. Kettlyne's experience of depression following the accident and her surgeries is fairly typical. She was more motivated initially to pursue therapy, but her attitude shifted as her treatment continued and her depression manifested.

Effect of PTSD on Mental Health

Individuals with PTSD experience several psychological difficulties or co-occurring disorders such as depression, anxiety disorders, and substance-use-related problems. Most people who experience significant past trauma struggle with one or more mental health and substance use disorders (Degenhardt et al., 2018 and Norman et al., 2018). It is estimated that over 50-66% of individuals diagnosed with PTSD also live with co-occurring addiction disorders.

PTSD and Depression

PTSD is characterized by indications such as anxiety, flashbacks, and reliving traumatic experiences that cause depression. People with depression display low mood, loss of interest and pleasure, and changes in energy levels. Research studies (Contractor et al., 2018) reveal that up to 6.8% of all people can develop both conditions. An example is PTSD and depression. An estimated 7.1% of the U.S. adult population experiences major depressive disorder (Contractor et al., 2018). They try to avoid talking or thinking about the event. Depression results in mood swings, negative thoughts, numbness, hopelessness, guilt, or self-loathing frequently.

PTSD and Anxiety Disorders

People with PTSD are in superior jeopardy of having anxiety disorders such as acute stress disorder, social anxiety disorder (SAD), panic disorder, and obsessive-compulsive disorder. Around 7% of men and 13% of women with PTSD also have panic disorder at the same period of time (Barbano et al., 2019).

Social Anxiety Disorder (SAD) and PTSD.

PTSD and SAD are co-related in several ways. People with PTSD face difficulties communicating or interacting with strangers or friends for fear of coming in contact with incident prompts, resulting in SAD development. Rates of people who experience SAD and PTSD range from 14% - 46% (McMillan et al., 2017).

Obsessive-Compulsive Disorder (OCD) and PTSD.

Studies by (Freire et al., 2020) indicate that between 4% – 22% of people with PTSD also have a diagnosis of obsessive-compulsive disorder (OCD). Conversely, 54% of people diagnosed with OCD reported having experienced one traumatic event in their entire lifetimes. These conditions make a person feel disordered, aggressive, and out of control, ultimately contributing to more anxiety and distress. In this situation, patients engage in activities such as isolation and avoidance to neutralize their behavior and overcome their anxiety from these distressing thoughts. Compulsive behaviors such as checking, ordering, or hoarding often makes them feel more controlled, secure, and less anxious. Individuals with traumatic OCD show more severe symptoms, e.g., suicidal thoughts, self-mutilation, panic disorder with agoraphobia, hoarding, compulsive spending. However, none of these self-reported behaviors are enough to make a formal diagnosis.

Panic Attacks and PTSD

The person diagnosed with PTSD commonly experiences recurrent and spontaneous panic attacks and flashbacks from their past traumatic experience (Richards et al., 2019). Panic attacks are characterized by feelings of intense horror that do not have a basis in reality. Panic attacks are often associated with physical vibrations, such as dizziness, nausea, and trembling. In addition, patients may experience heart palpitations, shortness of breath, and hot flashes upon being reminded of the traumatic event in the form of a nightmare or other memory.

Substance Use-Related Problems and PTSD

Research by Livingston et al. (2021) demonstrates a strong relationship between substance use issues and exposure to traumatic events. Usually, people who have experienced childhood physical abuse, criminal act, natural disasters, or other traumatic events turn to alcohol or drug misuse to help them deal with their emotional pain, bad memories, poor sleep, guilt, embarrassment, anxiety, fear, etc. Although anyone who underwent a traumatic experience can develop PTSD, people who already indulge in alcohol or drug use are more likely to experience traumatic events than those without these complications. According to studies conducted by Medscape, 21 - 43% of people who have PTSD also have a substance abuse problem. According to some findings (Krediet et al., 2020), drugs provide temporary relaxation and a release from terrifying memories. However, people might feel more alone when they're abusing drugs than during the phase of self-isolation. Furthermore, the reprieve is temporary. Drugs actually weaken the brain's functioning and are more likely to trigger the memories and impulses that make PTSD harder to control because drugs tend to intensify hallucinations and make recovery tougher.

Co-Occurring Conditions

- Suicidal thoughts
- Sleeping Problems
- Moral Injury: Damage done to an individual's moral conscience and values
- Neurocognitive Problems
- Anger and Violence
- Physical Problems

Conclusion

The research indicates that PTSD is a highly complex, disabling, and suffering disorder where people's past is always present for those who have been affected by traumatic events (Eisma et al., 2019). PTSD does not have a specific age limit and affects 1 out of every 11 persons. PTSD signifies a prospect for psychological and spiritual development because of the human ability to adjust and prosper despite experiencing adversity and tough times. However,

PTSD should be treated properly to prevent individuals from harming themselves and others.

Chapter 3
Mirror, Mirror

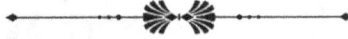

The mirror tells you everything. The mirror does not lie.

One of the most common challenges patients face during hospitalization is adjusting to hospital cooking. Portions are often small, and low-sodium restrictions make for bland and less-than-enjoyable meals. There is a logical reason for these limitations. For example, being served half of what a patient is used to may be part of specific nutritional requirements assigned to an individual. It's frustrating without counseling and education. There can be further disappointment when the food quality is inferior to what people are accustomed to. There can also be a lack of variety and even improper food temperatures. Substandard aesthetic appearance, or poor presentation, can result in patients not eating or eating less than anticipated. Patients are quick to realize that the hospital is not a place where the dining experience exceeds expectations.

I was advised by dieticians that after a few weeks, my taste buds would adjust and become sensitive to the taste of the food. As time passed, however, the day failed to arrive, and my taste buds began to scream for unique and appetizing home-cooked comfort food. Perhaps if Uber Eats or other online food ordering service had existed in 2001, I could have gotten away with accessing mouth-watering meals to satisfy my belly.

Cellphones in those days did not have internet access, at least no cellphone that I ever owned. Despite the absence of advanced technology, everyone I knew had a Nokia mobile device in their pocket in those days. Those little communication devices facilitated access to family members, friends, and co-workers. I was able to connect to people who brought me all kinds of foods. On days when more than one visitor arrived with a basket of goodies, I did not reject whatever surprise was in store for me, homemade or from a chain restaurant. Anything was better than the flavorless hospital food.

The daily routine for someone recuperating from orthopedic surgery in a hospital involves a little physical therapy, a little wound care, and a lot of cable television and even some people watching. Access to recreation, entertainment, and diversion is sparse. Therefore, visitors and the meals they brought were always a most welcome escape from the perpetually dull environment I was living in. I welcomed every person with a hug before my eyes went to the food. I had been spoiled. Being that I had always been a waif, going up a dress size or two was the last thing on my mind. In addition, being disappointed by repetitive surgeries and slow recovery, I had gotten into the habit of not looking at my legs or the rest of my body. This was a monumental mistake.

One fateful day, during a physical therapy session, I kindly asked the therapist to assist me to the bathroom to look at myself in front of the mirror. After months of being hospitalized, I suddenly felt like peeking. It was a spontaneous decision driven by curiosity.

The physical therapist wrapped a gait belt around my waist and transferred me from the bed to the walker. She assisted me to the bathroom. As I stood in front of the mirror, I did not recognize the person in the reflection. It could not possibly be me. The woman I was looking at had a great deal of cellulite and fat rolls. I had failed to notice the detrimental effect of excessive eating and the subsequent weight increase throughout my hospitalization. Since I was wearing a loose-fitting gown all the time, there was no waistband to call my attention to the significant problem. And given that I tended to bundle up under blankets when receiving guests, no one pointed out that I was gaining weight.

The food I coveted had become the bane of my existence. Medication was also part of the problem. Steroids, medication administered for wound healing and inflammation, can increase the appetite, alter the metabolism, and affect how the body distributes and deposits fat. I cursed myself for wallowing in my misery and failing to be conscious of what I had been doing to myself.

This weight was not healthy at all. It interfered with my recovery. Standing up shifted my weight downward, applying extreme pressure to the metal rods in my legs. Occasionally, it caused pain and bleeding. My physicians initially didn't notice the weight gain, but when they finally did, they were not pleased. It was recommended that I lose weight or continue to delay the recovery process and the possibility of ever walking again.

Looking at myself in front of a mirror was uncomfortable and heartbreaking. Where bandages and dressings pulled free, bone was visible. It was a sight that I would have preferred to avoid looking at ever again. But this was my world now.

I recalled all the injuries and deformities that I had witnessed throughout my career. Looking at my own body was very different than looking at patients with comparable conditions. This was my life. The nightmare was not coming to an end any time soon. I questioned whether I would ever return to good health.

That same day, I was blessed with the arrival of a roommate. I was fatigued often to the point of exhaustion at staring at the four walls of my room and the medical equipment that decorated them. Someone to interact with was wonderful. However, the roommate turned out to be morally bankrupt and thus a mockery and an insult to my personal situation.

I was paired with a drunk driver.

As soon as she revealed the reasons behind her injuries, I decided to cut the conversation short. I wished the staff would have put a little more thought into pairing me with someone who reminded me of why I was in the hospital. For the next few days, every time I spoke to the patient next to me, it brought on a host of negative emotions.

I am not the type of person who holds a grudge or tends to have conflictual social interactions with others. I should have felt sorry for my new neighbor, but I was angry and unhappy because of the unpleasant situation. It was upsetting that the young lady did not even recall getting into a vehicle. All she could remember was waking up inside the car wrapped around a tree. She survived the incident with a broken leg. She was in a reasonably stable enough condition that she might go home immediately after a minor procedure and the application of a cast.

I felt cheated, short-changed, that someone so reckless could have a better outcome than I, the responsible person with two jobs and a family. I was a decent person who followed the rules, wore my seatbelt, and paid bills on time. Yet, here I was, spending months in the hospital, dealing with extreme pain, while a person with an impaired driving history would be on her way home soon. It did not seem fair. I pulled the covers over my head and soon began to feel guilty for feeling that way, but that is what was going through my mind. I could not help it.

After so many weeks had passed, I noticed my husband's visits were growing further apart. He visited daily, then weekly, and now biweekly. Following the accident, when I was at the trauma center, he watched me undergo procedures, one after the other. He was very supportive and encouraging at the beginning, but as a rapid recovery did not manifest, and my body went through changes, I guess he could not handle it and lost hope. The debilitating condition I was in and the weight gain must have made me as unappealing to him as I had looked to myself. There were times he could not even look at me. My husband became less interested in my improvement and more distant. My husband eventually lost hope. He gave up on me.

I started feeling sorry for myself once more. My friends and family tried to lift my spirits. They kept reminding me of how blessed I was to be alive. However, I was wheelchair-bound, with little certainty I would walk again. I was feeling helpless, hopeless, and worthless. None of what they were saying really made me feel better because everyone returned to their normal lives at the end of the day, and I was still stuck in the hospital. Alone and frustrated, I would cry myself to sleep.

After the seemingly endless series of surgical procedures was finally done, it was time for me to be transferred from the hospital to a rehabilitation center. I had undergone a total of six surgeries. The rehabilitation center was also part nursing home and housed numerous elderly residents. The staff informed me I was the youngest patient ever to be admitted to their facility. It was unsettling to think that they had minimal experience providing care to a patient my age.

This new facility was not as effective as the hospital in helping me with an exercise regimen that improved my functional abilities. The sense of confinement or isolation was no different. Sometimes time passed at a snail's pace, sometimes it seemed to stand still, and sometimes it seemed to be moving backward. Not surprisingly, the food was no better. I knew I needed to eat fruits, grains, vegetables, and lean protein, but the food was atrocious. Understandably, when preparing meals for a geriatric population, soft and mushy nutrients must be expected to accommodate those who cannot chew or digest solid food. It was so bad that I refused to eat the meals. However, my mother lived nearby and was gracious enough to prepare salads for me.

I cannot say the three-month stay at the rehab was a completely horrible experience. But I could have done without the inconsistencies in the delivery of services, especially the wound care that was ordered to be performed three times a day. Due to the severity of my injuries and wounds, I did not have the option of receiving home health care. What made it all tolerable, what helped me keep my sanity, were frequent visits from my friends and co-workers. My mother visited almost every day of the week.

My husband only visited about three times, once a month. I tried to be positive, polite, and funny, but it always seemed as if he was in a rush to get to work or run an errand. He called perhaps once a week for a few minutes but seemed to be distracted or unconcerned. I took it as a sign that he no longer wanted to be in a relationship. I kept this pain bottled up inside me. I never shared it with anyone. With the scheduled release date inching closer, I had faith that the mental anguish my husband was going through could be worked out. The only difficulty was that I planned to live with my mother and stepfather while my husband was staying with his family across town. It would be difficult to find a private place to talk, but not impossible. Whenever tears welled up in my eyes in the presence of a visitor, I used my injuries and emotional trauma as an excuse.

Before leaving the rehab, the orthopedic surgeon ordered a seventh and final surgical procedure. The last thing I wanted was to undergo another operation. I was tired and overwhelmed. I could not take it anymore. When he left, I started to cry and asked God why I was enduring so much agony. After giving the situation some thought and believing I had the strength to recover independently, I planned on refusing the procedure. I did not know it at the time, and I would not be privy to the details until later that there would be no more invasive or reconstructive operations. Only skin grafts were necessary. Of course, there are inherent risks and the potential for complications with any surgery, but I could emotionally handle skin grafts.

As mentioned, the details of the surgery were not yet made clear to me. Physical therapy and wound care were still taking place. Once a week, an ambulance van transported me to hyperbaric wound treatment. And a different ambulance van shuttled me to follow-up appointments at the orthopedic surgeon's office at a nearby outpatient center. On one of those routine trips, while I was waiting for the return ride to the rehab center, I met a woman waiting for her ride in front of the outpatient center. Her belongings fell to the ground. My son was with me, and I asked him to pick up the items. He playfully took his time, picking up one item at a time, running back and forth. I began to get irritated watching him. Then I realized he wanted to make the endeavor last. I could appreciate his boredom, and I could see my son was just trying to entertain himself as best he could. The woman was amused by his antics, and it provided an opportunity for us to introduce ourselves and speak to one another.

She thanked him for his help, made small talk, and looked at me with curiosity. The woman asked what had happened to my legs and how I was doing.

To needlessly avoid evoking pity from people I met and interacted with, I always responded with courage. Sometimes I gave people a brief, positive response, sometimes I shared a smile, a nod, and a thumb's up. I always tried to make little of the entire ordeal.

My new acquaintance was not convinced. "I can see something is bothering you," she commented.

I really did not want to share anything with a stranger. But I figured I would never see this woman again, so what the heck.

I revealed the cause of my injuries and expressed how tired I was from the endless surgeries. I communicated that I was feeling frustrated because another surgical procedure had been scheduled. This one would be the seventh operation.

The woman looked over my shoulder into the sky. She returned her gaze, and with a smile, she said, "Baby, you go ahead and have that surgery."

"I know, I know," I grumbled, "but I am just so tired of it all."

"You know what?" she asserted, "Let me tell you a little something about myself: I'm on a 24-hour watch. Do you know what it means to be on a 24-hour watch?"

"No," I responded, interested in an explanation. I was not familiar with that phrase.

"I was diagnosed with cancer and was placed on a 24-hour watch five years ago," she revealed. "My whole body is cancerous except for my heart."

I could not believe my ears — her healthcare team was closely monitoring her condition because she could die at any moment. And there I was, feeling sorry for myself once more when someone was much worse off.

The woman explained how she refused to allow self-pity to get the best of her despite the terminal prognosis. With a laugh, she added, "I am going to live every day to the fullest because every day could be my last."

I was speechless, and all I could do was nod.

"So, you go ahead and have that surgery. There is still hope for you."

For a few seconds, she succeeded in shaming and humbling me. Of course, she was right, but I had a lot of issues I had to deal with. I needed to find a new home and purchase a used car. I also had marital issues sitting too long on the back burner. With a shake of my head, I believe I acknowledged what I thought was an affirmative response, but it was likely not too convincing.

The woman proclaimed, "Give it a chance. One day you will walk across the field at your child's football game."

My transport van pulled up. I thanked her and wished her good health. There was a brief exchange of pleasantries before the ambulance van driver wheeled me into position and secured the door. My son was still chatting with her through an open window as we pulled away. I was relieved I would not have to pretend she had convinced me to undergo another procedure.

I never saw the woman again but often wondered what became of her. At the time, her sage advice was, to say the least, not what I wanted. However, the brief encounter gave me hope, and I did have the surgery when I learned it was only a skin graft.

Within the week, I was re-admitted to the hospital for the final procedure. It would be a short three-day stay while nurses evaluated my post-operative status. I would be allowed to receive outpatient physical therapy and wound care at my mother's home. After so many months, I was very close to being liberated from the confines of healthcare facilities. Instead of being thrilled and overjoyed, I did not feel relief, and I was not getting adequate rest. The last few days, the final hours, were agonizingly long.

On my last day in the hospital, I experienced a delayed adverse reaction to morphine. This was not the first time I had received that specific pain medication. Therefore, I did not think it was the cause of the itching that I began to feel during a bed bath. I thought the nurse was using the wrong soap and let her know. She did not take my comment lightly. She was offended and reacted by stepping back and taking a defensive posture before handing me the washcloth and telling me in a stern tone that I could finish the job on my own since she was not doing a good job.

I was taken aback. That was no way to speak to a patient. My suggestion was not a criticism. I merely verbalized a clear and legitimate concern. Had I been a frail and defenseless geriatric patient, the authoritative body language, the strong words, and the cross facial expression would have intimidated and frightened me. Good bedside manner requires that healthcare professionals express empathy toward the patients under their care. A caring connection promotes trust as patients feel valued and respected.

Unfortunately, the lack of decency and professionalism that I used to witness from time to time as an employee was something I experienced with greater frequency laying in a hospital bed. Whether one is a physician, nurse, or respiratory therapist, passing a test does not make a good healthcare worker. Incivility is often chalked up to workplace pressures, facility culture, low morale, or any number of excuses that attempt to justify the words and acts of employees as an isolated incident that align with the values of the facility. However, it cannot be denied that some people are just not meant to be at the bedside.

I reported the incident to the department director, who quickly responded. The nurse had no idea that I had once been employed by the hospital. She tried to apologize and expressed that had she known, she would have treated me differently.

The feeble apology made me more upset. I was not seeking favorable treatment, just humane treatment. After all, I was a patient in need, and no patient deserves to be treated with rudeness.

The annoyance was infuriating. I chose to remain silent and gave her a nod to acknowledge her attempt to pacify my ire. I was so glad to be getting out of the facility soon because I was at the end of my rope regarding patience and understanding.

Research: Distorted Body Image

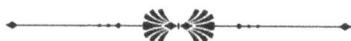

Tragic experiences leading to physical changes really do not help with coping and recovering. Kettlyne's physical body had transformed, and it had taken a physiological, emotional, and mental toll on her. However, body image is a complicated concept and consists of self-perceptions, cognitions, emotions, and behaviors that one holds toward own physical characteristics (Ryding & Kuss, 2020). According to Mountford & Koskina (2015), body image disturbance is an altered belief that an individual perceives about their body weight or shape. It incorporates the undue influence of negative assumptions, feelings, and a sense of embodiment about the appearance of the body. However, body image also stems from what the mirror reflects about the person. It can also be influenced by various social and environmental factors such as culture and media, both negatively and positively. Distorted body image and body dissatisfaction are painful in both clinical and non-clinical populations of the United States and cause a significant negative impact on psychological and physical wellbeing.

The National Eating Disorder Association (NEDA) explores an array of beliefs, experiences, and generalizations that affect a person's social life, self-confidence, and temperaments that ultimately result in persistent anxiety and low self-esteem. Devrim et al. (2018) research reveals that a distorted body image, also known as negative body image, and in severe cases can lead to multiple eating disorders and body dysmorphic disorder (BDD).

Studies have found that eating disorders associated with distorted body image are more commonly seen in women than men (Gorrell & Murray, 2019). These misperceptions such as body attractiveness, health, acceptability, and functionality originate from early childhood and become a solid pillar with age and feedback from friends and family members. Friends, family, and relatives reinforce many misperceptions due to the conditioning of social expectation.

Perfectionism and self-criticism can also influence the progress of the body's negative image to distortion. Typically, people begin believing in perceptions and feelings than actual appearance. For instance, a person experiencing bulimia sees their waist in the mirror as wider than the actual size. Psychotherapists and mental health professionals can help address these body image concerns, develop tactics for managing insecurities, and improve emotional and physical health.

Below, we explore the concept of distorted body image. The factors that contribute to negative body image, symptoms of syndromes and eating disorders, the effect of negative body image on physical and psychological health, how to assess own and other's body image along with strategies for improving it, and the proportion of dissatisfied American teens, men, and women about their body image.

Concept and History Perception of Distorted Body Image

According to the findings of Thompson & Schaefer (2019), body image is a multidimensional concept and is defined as a subjective image of individuals, especially beliefs about one's physical appearance and feelings, regardless of what their actual body looks like. Moreover, it encompasses a collection of past experiences created in the cerebral sensory cortex. Over the past century, a wide range of neurologists proposed various models, including genetic, neuroscientific, cognitive-behavioral, sociocultural, and feminist, to understand the concept of body image.

In 1935, Paul Schilder, an Austrian neurologist, and psychoanalyst proposed a biopsychosocial approach and coined the term "body image" in his famous book, *The Image, and Appearance of the*

Human Body. According to the book, body image focuses on depersonalization's experiences in individuals with schizophrenia which is the detachment within oneself where the individual views the world through a vague and dreamlike lens. They feel like they are outside of reality looking in and that there is very little significance to the world. (Szczotka & Majchrowicz, 2018).

On the other hand, there is a theory of unique body experiences in amputees known as "phantom limb syndrome." Hilde Bruch was the first to recognize body image distortion as central to the psychopathology of eating disorders in 1962 (Murnen & Smolak, 2019). The research explored that body image is a self-motivated phenomenon that alters with age, attitude, and clothing. Another study classified body image as the illustration of identity derived from external and internal body experiences. Bailey & Gammage (2019) noted that body image is a multifaceted construct comprising thoughts, feelings, assessments, and actions related to one's physical body.

Factors Contributing to Negative Body Image

In this modern era, many people are experiencing body dissatisfaction. Some people may be bullied about their appearance in their childhood. In contrast, others grow in a household where parents actively promote weight control activities to be slim, particularly in teenage girls and women, who emphasize ideal body size and appearances more. However, the family is responsible for helping to develop the body image, body size, attitudes, and eating patterns of their children at an early age. Parents can direct their children toward a positive self-image or increase the distorted body image and eating concerns.

Indirect parental behaviors, including parents' negative comments about their child's body structure and weight, can lead to self-criticism. On the other hand, BMI, society, television, social media, and low self-esteem can also contribute to a distorted body image. Additional factors that play a significant role in a negative body image include culture, psyche, gender, age, marital status, and education level.

Body Mass Index (BMI) and Self-Esteem

BMI is a biological component and is one of the most significant factors influencing body image and body satisfaction (Gentile et al., 2018). The BMI measurement is considered a reliable indicator of body fat percentage for most people. It measures the body fat based on the height and weight of a person and helps screen for possible health problems related to high body fat levels.

Several reports show that overweight individuals are more susceptible to fear associated with being criticized. This state of negativity adversely impacts their mental health and increases their rate of depression due to lower self-esteem. Higher self-esteem works as a shielding factor, reducing the level of anxiety caused by others' unfavorable judgments. Self-esteem is more influential in racial, ethnic, and gender groups, placing a high regard on physical appearance.

Society, Mass Media, and Media

Social acceptance is a serious component of our lives and a societal phenomenon that influences women and men to maintain ideal body shapes considered socially desirable. To fulfill the requirements for social acceptance, people tend to develop behavioral responses, including dieting and gaining muscles, which boost their social desirability, particularly in adolescents. And hence, this pressure significantly contributes to negative body perceptions and body dissatisfaction.

More than ever, our youth and teenagers today are bombarded by diverse forms of mass media, including television, movies, videos, billboards, magazines, music, newspapers, the internet, and social media, which have the greatest impact. The desire for the ideal muscular body in males and a slim physique in females directly correlates with media advertisements, film stars, and images. Media factors influence psychological conditions, body image misperception, body dissatisfaction, and eating disorders.

Effect of Negative Body Image on Individual's Health

A negative body image may lead to self-destructive behaviors and psychological health problems (Radziwiłłowicz & Lewandowska, 2017). For Kettlyne, this occurred after months of limited activity, a modified diet, and steroids. Still, negative body images can also result from less significant physical changes or even none at all. Distorted body image can affect self-esteem, mood, capabilities, and social and occupational functioning. These misperceptions are frequently seen in America's general population and proved as an essential factor that causes serious illnesses such as BDD, anorexia nervosa, and bulimia nervosa.

Also, dissatisfaction with the body can lead to several physically and emotionally unhealthy habits such as eating limitations, especially among teenagers. In addition, individuals who are enormously unhappy with their bodies have a greater risk of developing muscle dysmorphia, relationship problems, and self-harm tendencies. Recent research on the effects of distorted body image elucidates that negative body image can also cause life-threatening disorders such as Obsessive-compulsive disorder (OCD), Social anxiety disorder (SAD), and major depressive disorder.

Body Dysmorphic Disorder

Body Dysmorphia is a severe mental health disorder. BDD people become obsessed with thinking about one or more perceived defects or flaws in their appearance (Sandgren & Lavallee, 2018). It may be a small flaw such as a crooked nose, an uneven smile, or larger/smaller eyes – traits that may seem minor or unremarkable by others. But the individual feels embarrassed, ashamed, and anxious about their imperfections, leading them to avoid many social situations. Their unpleasant thoughts and fear can cause severe emotional distress and interfere with their daily functioning, such as missing work or school and isolating themselves, even from family and friends. BDD is mutually caused by environmental, psychological, and biological factors. Bullying and teasing may substitute the feelings of inadequacy, shame, and fear of ridicule. Though, family history of BDD, the abnormal release of chemicals in the brain, personality traits, and bad life experiences equally cause BDD.

Symptoms of BDD

There are two primary symptoms of BDD:

1) Appearance preoccupations
2) Repetitive, compulsive behavior

Appearance Preoccupations

Individuals with BDD can become obsessed with any part of their body, believing that their body parts look ugly or abnormal. It normally affects common areas of the face, which are readily visible – nose, complexion, wrinkles, acne, blemishes, hair (how it looks, the length, whether it is thinning or balding). But they can also focus on skin, chest and muscle size, stomach, and genitalia.

Repetitive Compulsive Behaviors

According to (Giraldo-O'Meara & Belloch, 2018), BDD appearance preoccupations fuel repetitive, compulsive behaviors. People use these behaviors to fix, hide, inspect, or obtain reassurance about the disliked body parts. These unusual behaviors may include:

- Camouflaging – constantly adjusting one's clothing to hide disliked body parts
- Comparing
- Mirror checking
- Excessive grooming
- Reassurance seeking/questioning of others
- Skin picking
- Clothes changing
- Tanning
- Excessive exercising or weight lifting
- Unnecessary shopping
- Seeking cosmetic surgery, dermatologic treatment, or other cosmetic procedures
- Social anxiety and avoidance
- Suicidal thoughts

Eating Disorders

In the literature review of Kostecka et al. (2019), distorted body image is a strong predictor of eating disorders caused by genetic or environmental factors. In this type of mental health disorder, people may intensely inspect their bodies and tie their worth to a specific appearance, working to attain an ideal size. The negative behavior of self-evaluation excessively influenced by body shape and weight is consistent with a diagnosis of either anorexia nervosa or bulimia nervosa. Moreover, they focus on perceived flaws rather than their entire appearance, such as emphasizing a soft stomach while ignoring their visible ribs.

Anorexia Nervosa

Anorexia nervosa is a common eating disorder that cannot be taken lightly because it can be a potentially life-threatening psychiatric disorder. It has the highest mortality rate of any mental illness in America. Those with this condition believe themselves to be overweight even when the reverse is true. They often severely restrict their food intake and engage in various behaviors to reduce weight, including excessive exercise, vomiting after eating, and the routine use of laxatives.

Physical, Behavioral, and Emotional Symptoms of Anorexia Nervosa

- **Physical:** Abdominal pain, anemia, bruising easily, brittle nails, cold hands and feet, constipation, lanugo (downy hair all over the body), loss of hair on the scalp, extreme dehydration, fainting, osteoporosis, pale skin, abnormal menstrual period cycle in females, low blood pressure and heart rate, muscle loss, and weakness.

- **Behavioral:** Complaining about stomachache, denial of hunger, desperate to exercise, unusual eating behavior, fatigue, fear of gaining weight or being fat, and may hide foods to avoid eating them.

- **Emotional:** Anxiety, depression, low self-esteem, easily annoyed, self-critical, and ☐little or no motivation to engage in relationships.

Bulimia Nervosa and Symptoms

Bulimia nervosa is an eating disorder characterized by binge-purge cycles. A person with bulimia frequently eats large amounts of food in a specific period until their stomach becomes painfully full, followed by purging via inducing vomiting or misuse of laxatives.

The symptoms of bulimia may include:

- Bloodshot eyes
- Chest pains
- Chronic bouts of constipation
- Electrolyte imbalances
- Dehydration
- Sore throat
- Headache
- Lightheadedness
- Mouth ulcers
- Stomach aches
- Vomiting blood
- Compensatory purging
- Use of drugs or detox teas to suppress appetite
- Social withdrawal
- Depression

- Extreme irritability

- Self-critical

- Out-of-control emotions

- Excessive exercise

- Excessive fasting

Assessment of Distorted Body Image

Evaluating one's and another's body image involves two independent modalities, i.e., an attitudinal component and a perceptual component.

Gauging the Attitudinal Component

A variety of psychometric tools and techniques are used to evaluate body dissatisfaction. There are numerous quantifiable procedures available for body image assessment in children, adolescents, and adults. However, figure rating scales containing figures that vary in body size are the most helpful assessment tools.

The attitudinal component of body image in children can be evaluated using multiple measurement techniques: Kid's Eating Disorders Survey, Body Image Assessment Procedure for Children's (BIA-C), Body Image Scale, and Body-Esteem Questionnaire.

The attitudinal component involves the feelings that an individual possesses about their body size and shape. Measurements presented for assessing the attitudinal component of body image in adolescents and adults are:

- Contour Drawing Rating Scale

- Multidimensional Body-Self Relations Questionnaire (MBSRQ)

- Body Image Assessment (BIA)

- Somatomorphic Matrix

- Body Esteem Scale

- Body-Image Ideals Questionnaire (BIQ)

- Self-Image Questionnaire for Young Adolescents (SIQYA)

- Attention to Body Shape Scale (ABS).

Gauging the Perceptual Component

Researchers believe that evaluating the perceptual component of distorted body image has been proved as more complex and challenging than the attitudinal component. Two general groups along with methods have been developed:

Depictive Methods

The participant compares and contrasts their body image with a visual or a 2D image in this method, such as the distorted photograph technique, video distortion, and template matching.

Metric Methods

In this method, participants compare their body shape to a physical length or 1D standard using instruments such as the moving caliper, the image marking procedure, or an adjustable light beam apparatus.

Computer Generated Imagery (CGI)

This method has been relatively recently adopted in the world of measuring perceptual components of body image. It is used to create standard stimuli or personalized 3D avatars that reflect body shape changes based on BMI.

Strategies and Techniques for Improving Body Image

According to de Freitas et al. (2018), a body image does not develop in isolation but is influenced by norms, the fashion industry, and surroundings. Fortunately, researchers have formulated strategies and techniques that may help people feel more positive about their bodies and minimize the consequences of this mental disorder.

- Spend time with those who possess a positive outlook
- Avoid offending media and comparison
- Encourage and practice positive self-talk
- Wear comfortable clothes that look good on you without hesitation
- Have a nutritious diet
- Meditate regularly

Cognitive-Behavioral Therapy (CBT)

CBT is an intervention that targets cognitive and behavioral procedures and helps individuals to modify dysfunctional thoughts and actions about their body image.

Techniques that help to Enhance Physical Fitness

These interventions comprise aerobic or anaerobic exercises that support individuals in enhancing physical capacities like muscular strength and encouraging them to emphasize functionality rather than appearance.

Statistics

The vast majority – over 91% – of American women are dissatisfied with their body shape and size (Moreno-Domínguez et al., 2018).

Over 58% of teenage girls were found to have engaged in weight controlling activities to achieve an ideal body shape (Fung et al., 2019). Similarly, only 5% of American women naturally possess the body type often depicted on television (Mastro & Figueroa-Caballero, 2018). Furthermore, one in every three people involved in pathological dieting, and one in every four suffered from a partial or full-on eating disorder. The results of one survey indicate that more than 40% of women and approximately 20% of men have shown a desire for cosmetic surgery regardless of gender, age, marital status, and race (Greenberg et al., 2019).

The prevalence rate of anorexia nervosa is about 0.48% of girls aged 15 – 19. Regarding bulimia nervosa, about 1%-5% of adolescent girls meet the criteria (Kantha, Rani, Parameswaran, & Indira, 2016).

In addition to this, adolescent boys and girls are at greater risk of low self-esteem and depression, possibly leading to early sexual activities, substance abuse, and suicidal thoughts (Manaf, 2016). According to the International Society of Aesthetic Plastic Surgery findings, approximately 8% - 15% of individuals with BDD search for plastic surgery, and 90% of people who get cosmetic surgery develop worse symptoms due to dissatisfaction with the surgery outcomes (Greenberg et al., 2019). Moreover, the suicide rate among people with BDD is 45 times higher than that of the general U.S population (Watson & Ban, 2021).

Conclusion

Body image dissatisfaction is a severe health problem. A higher level of body dissatisfaction is associated with an inferior quality of life, emotional distress, and an elevated risk of the severe syndrome and eating disorders. It refers to negative evaluations of one's body when somebody perceives discrepancies between their actual body and ideal body. Directing mindfulness-based treatments can help foster a willingness to accept the present state and cultivate compassion. However, additional efforts are required to build and promote a positive body image, supporting good physical health and psychological wellbeing. Distorted body image and associated judgmental behaviors that led to adverse health-related outcomes should be recognized and provided with various treatment approaches to address this devastating health problem. Doing so will help improve a person's quality of life by helping them achieve higher wellness levels.

Chapter 4
Survivor's Guilt

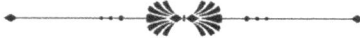

———————— ❧❧ ————————

The day arrived when I was finally discharged from the hospital to continue physical therapy and wound care at home. Although I was still wheelchair-bound with orthopedic hardware on my lower extremities, a physical therapist would provide daily exercise. Because of the physical restrictions, a home health nurse would visit routinely to administer various prescribed medications such as Lovenox, an anticoagulant that helps prevent the formation of blood clots. There were no longer exposed bones due to the recent skin graft surgery. Significant progress had been made regarding wound healing, but there would still be visits by wound care nurses three times a week.

My mother was a tremendous help throughout the transition from the hospital to her home. She hired someone to assist me with activities of daily living while she was at work. My mother would relieve the private aide in the evenings and help take care of my son and me.

My basic needs, meals, bathing, and dressing were met, but my hair was unkempt. My braids had started to lock and needed to come out. My mother recommended that I make a hair salon appointment and get the job done. I was mostly restricted to the wheelchair, but I could get around a little using a walker. Nonetheless, my mother insisted that I demonstrate my current ability to ambulate. I showed her that, with the help of a walker, I could take five small steps. The effort was painful. It was a strain and a struggle, but I was committed to having my hair done, so I held a big smile throughout the demonstration to put my mother at ease. I was excited to go to the salon because grooming had been the last thing on my mind during my hospitalization. This would be the first hair appointment since the accident all those months ago. Now, back in civilization, getting my hair done would not only boost my self-esteem but would also represent my first step toward normalcy.

I went to the hair appointment on a Thursday. I remember the day of the week because it was my mother's payday. Sitting in the salon chair felt strange but comfy. The experience gave me flashbacks of my senior prom and my wedding, two times in which I needed to look like a fancier version of myself. Today was not supposed to be a milestone moment. I just wanted to feel like I did before the accident. And it worked. I felt like a million bucks. There was something about having one's hair washed and conditioned that was restful, relaxing, and rejuvenating.

After the visit to the salon, I waited for my mother to pick me up and the agreed-upon time. She did not show up. We did not have cellphones to text in those days, but we did have beepers. I paged my mother, but she failed to respond. It was unusual for her not to return a page. The only thing I could do was continue to page her every half hour and hope she would answer. Afternoon turned into evening, and there was no return call. I was stuck at the salon and very worried. What was going on?

As I was working up the courage to hobble to a bus stop, my sixteen-year-old brother arrived with a friend who was old enough to drive. I asked my brother what happened. He told me our stepfather had sent them to pick me up because our mother was in the hospital. My heart sank. Something bad had happened.

The distance between the salon and the hospital could not have been more than a handful of miles. The trip took no more than ten minutes, but it seemed far longer as we were caught behind one red light after another.

Stepping out of the vehicle at the hospital, I was met by a friend of the family who informed me that my mother complained of a headache at work before collapsing. Her colleagues did not even have time to bring a chair. Fire rescue was called, and my mother was rushed to the nearest hospital for emergency care.

My brother got me into the facility using a courtesy wheelchair. I was able to speak to the ER physician, who advised that diagnostic imaging tests revealed my mother had suffered a brain aneurysm. When a blood vessel in the brain ruptures, the blood spills into the brain cavity compressing the organ. The physician was considering drilling a burr hole into my mother's head to help relieve the pressure, but my mother was unresponsive by then. Her current systolic blood pressure was above 250 mmHg, and her diastolic blood pressure was above 140 mmHg. These are life-threatening blood pressure levels. Intravenous medication had not been able to lower her blood pressure, and no medical intervention would likely be able to restore her to consciousness. Shortly after that, my mother was placed on life-support.

I recalled reading that studies on the electrical activity in the brain had been done on people in the dying process, and there was a possibility that responses to sounds occurred even during an unconscious state. It gave me comfort to sit at my mother's side, hold her hand, and whisper in her ear how much I loved her. I asked the physician to explain the prognosis in simple terms so that she could understand what was going on with her. He obliged and expressed that my mother's chances of survival were slim. Consenting to drill the burr hole was a difficult decision to make.

My brother stayed in the waiting room surrounded by my mother's friends and colleagues. My brother was young and impressionable, and I did not want his last memories of our mother to be one in which she was lying on a stretcher with machines keeping her alive. As the older child and as a healthcare worker with a reasonable understanding of the situation, making the decisions was my responsibility.

My mother had been nurturing, giving, and loving to my brother and me throughout her life. She demonstrated limitless energy, multi-tasked with her eyes closed, worked long hours, and barely got any rest making sure our homework was done. During my hospitalization and rehab, my mother was the one person I could count on to listen to my doubts and fears.

After so much time, just when the chaos and craziness were coming to an end, the woman who was my rock was now lying on a stretcher in critical condition. I felt frustrated, overwhelmed, my mind reeling while desperately trying to cope. I wanted to tell her I was sorry for putting her through so much stress due to my injuries. Never in a million years had I thought that it would come to this. So sudden. I was ashamed of all the clichéd clutter that littered my brain.

The long day and my physical limitations were taking a toll. My strength was failing. I was physically and emotionally devastated and exhausted. It was so hard to leave my mother's side. I felt that if I could just stay near her, time would not advance, and her life-threatening condition would not deteriorate. I put my hand on her cheek, closed my eyes, and thought about the good times. Each beep of the cardiac monitor gave me an extra second of hope, but I knew her purposeful life would soon begin to fade. Due to the extensive damage, I opted not to consent to the procedure. I felt it would only prolong her misery.

My dear brother escorted me home, both of us utterly overcome with grief. We did not speak about what had happened because acknowledging that our mother was going to die seemed like we were abandoning her. No sooner than we arrived at home, I received a telephone call from the hospital to notify me that my mother had gone into respiratory arrest and passed away. My mother's precious light had been extinguished. I drew an uneasy breath and tried to call out to my brother but felt the weight of the world begin to press down upon me. My eyes became two incessant fountains releasing hot tears of frustration and anger. I clenched my fists and muttered, "This is all my fault."

With my face buried in my hands, I thought about all the terrible things that had happened since the day my house burned down. I raised my eyes to heaven to say a prayer. Instead, I questioned God, "Lord, how could I have the gift to help save the lives of so many people but not be able to help my mother?"

Feelings of guilt devastated me.

My mother had been diagnosed with hypertension, and she was prescribed medication for the condition. My mother was adherent to her treatment regimen. She ate properly and was not overweight. She had been doing quite well throughout the years. However, perhaps if my mother had not been so involved with my care, she would have been able to avoid stress, find the time to exercise, or do something that could have helped spare her life.

Before my injury, I was an EMT technician, a first responder. I was trained to recognize the signs of an emergency. Granted, brain aneurysms are sudden and have a very poor prognosis. And I also realize that high blood pressure, as radio and television ads uphold, is the silent killer. Nevertheless, had my life not become so complicated, there may have been something I could have done to help my mother improve her health.

As much as I wanted to wallow in my pain, I could not allow myself to indulge in self-pity. Now that my mother was gone, it was up to me to care for my teenage brother. He would look to me for guidance, and I had to be strong for him.

My mother's twin sister was living in New York at the time, and when she heard the news, she immediately flew to Florida to make funeral arrangements. Her assistance was most welcome. After the funeral, I returned to my stepfather's home. He had taken my mother's passing hard. After a few days of bereavement, my stepfather declared he was going to start charging my brother and me rent. He claimed that before my mother died, they discussed this issue. I found that very hard to believe. Neither my brother nor I were employed. He was still in high school, and I was still physically impaired. We had no way to pay rent. My mother would never have agreed to this. Once again, I found myself between a rock and a hard place.

The only option I had was to reach out to Sally. I explained what had happened and asked if I could stay at her house. Being the loyal friend that she was, Sally welcomed my son, my brother, and myself into her home.

My husband was not in the picture. He failed to show up to the funeral. He was no longer involved in the lives of his wife and son.

Research: Bereavement

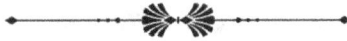

The same year she lost her house and had a life-changing car accident, Kettlyne lost her mother. Talk about pouring salt on an open wound. The pain of losing a loved one is challenging under the best of circumstances, and these were certainly far from the best for her.

According to Neimeyer (2019), people face a high degree of fragmentation in physical and mental health that results from bereavement. Experiencing a loved one's death is highly stressful, especially when it comes accidentally or prematurely. It significantly shakes the relational world's foundations and challenges grief-stricken sufferers to find meaning in the loss and its aftermath. Everyone reacts differently. Some people ultimately adjust to their loss fairly quickly without seeking professional psychological intervention, whereas others take a year or longer to manage.

In contrast, bereavement is the period of grief and mourning associated with detriments in physical health such as problems sleeping, severe illness, loss of appetite, and multiple psychological issues such as anger, guilt, anxiety, sadness, and despair. There is even an elevated risk of mortality for those suffering bereavement, mainly in the early weeks and months after sudden loss (Trevino et al., 2018). The duration of the mourning phase and the vulnerability of bereaved individuals depend upon how attached the person was to the deceased.

The time between death and the funeral or memorial, burial, and cremation highly influenced mourning intensity. However, how people mourn is also influenced by personal, familial, cultural, religious perspectives, and societal beliefs. Here we aim to summarize and discuss the current knowledge about grief and various psycho-social responses to types of bereavement and when to seek help.

Types of Bereavements

It is estimated that the reactions to death do not follow a specific set of patterns but vary by the relationship with the deceased. For example, experiencing a spouse's death is different from the death of a child or parent. However, types of bereavements along with the life cycle possess diverse manifestations. Furthermore, it holds implications for the health of an individual through possible associations with morbidity and mortality.

Spousal Bereavement

Experiencing a spouse's death is an emotionally devastating event and generally is recognized as the most stressful of all possible losses. The strength and persistence of the pain associated with the emotional value of matrimonial promises connect spouses. Following the loss of a spouse, a single parent can be susceptible to overload and emotional collapse with the added burden of sole responsibility for children and unfamiliar tasks to be accomplished in addition to accustomed ones. On losing their sex partners, many widows lost interest in sex as one aspect of their grief (Carr, 2020). Additionally, they often experience anhedonia (inability to feel pleasure), feelings of exclusion from couples' sociability, trouble in establishing new relationships, and social isolation. Some bereaved widows successfully adapt to their new living conditions, but others suffer from long-lasting emotional problems.

Perinatal Bereavement

Perinatal bereavement afflicts parents who experience their infant's death (Boyle et al., 2020). Death may occur in several ways, such as miscarriage, stillbirth, elective termination, or the death of an older child.

This type of grief is characterized by a multifaceted emotional response, commonly as distress in parents, and may be influenced by internal and external factors. Mourning occurs as an intense expression of loss and is influenced by culture, religion, and tradition. However, bereavement support interventions, such as creating souvenirs, naming the deceased baby, holding the baby, and performing a funeral service, may reduce the degree and length of the grief response during perinatal bereavement.

When it comes to older children, it can have more serious emotional effects because the child has lived longer, and there are more memories of the child. It is predicted that 400,000 children under the age of 25 die each year due to accidents, diseases, suicide, or murder, leaving over 800,000 bereaved parents in America (Stevenson et al., 2016).

Parental Bereavement

This type of grief is associated with the loss of a parent in adulthood, which is what Kettlyne experienced. According to Apelian and Nesteruk (2017), 5% of America's adult citizens lost their parents within a year. In modern-day Western society, losing a parent in adulthood is less disruptive, although it still causes intense grief reactions (and if the adult is situationally dependent upon the parent, such as Kettlyne was, the effects can be more intense).

Simultaneously, some studies demonstrate an increased tendency to thoughts of suicide and rates of attempted suicide and depression. Moreover, data from Apelian and Nesteruk (2017) suggest that adults mourn the death of nurturing caretakers very severely – exhibiting stronger emotional reactions to a mother compared to a father's death. However, generally, the loss of a parent in adulthood was the least disruptive and caused the least intense grief reactions, perhaps because it is the most normative loss. Some adults show an increased rate of the consumption of sedatives or alcohol. However, most get back to their busy life after a few days.

Death of a Sibling Bereavement

Siblings' grief is often ignored. There is an absence of a record of losing siblings because less impact has been observed than the death of a spouse, child, or parent. Most siblings do not live together or are likely to have social contact with them. However, some comments suggested that many sisters and brothers continue to visit each other, share memories, plan reunions, manage responsibility for aging parents, and psychologically influence each other explicitly or implicitly, particularly in selecting marital partners. Sibling death in childhood may be challenging to resolve and could complicate grief reactions. The anxiety following a sibling's death may be particularly acute among the elderly as it aggravates fear of one's own impending death.

Suicide Bereavement

The recent finding of Scocco et al. (2020) called this type of grief a "personal and interpersonal disaster" because suicide or homicide of a family member or close friend results in devastating response and bereavement. Every year, over 27,000 people commit suicide in the United States. Men are three times more vulnerable than women, and whites are nearly twice as likely as blacks to experience this (Miron et al., 2019).

Moreover, survivors of suicide experienced longer-lasting physical and mental health problems than bereaved individuals from other causes of death. Indeed, one study (Perng & Renz, 2018) shows an increased mortality rate among the widowed whose spouses committed suicide. In addition, children whose parents committed suicide are at risk for enduring suicidal consequences (Burrell et al., 2018).

About Bereavement and When to Seek Help

Bereavement is characterized by grief that holds a range of emotions in individuals when experiencing someone special's death. As a result, people adopt different ways to deal with grief. Some seek comfort with friends and family members, while some take weeks, months, or even years to work through their bereavement.

Symptoms

Grief causes a varied number of symptoms and affects people in different ways. Some of the most common symptoms are shock and numbness, overwhelming sadness—with crying, tiredness, exhaustion, and anger—toward the person responsible for the loss, and guilt. Other symptoms include social isolation, loss of enjoyment, fear of establishing new relationships, hurting oneself, sudden changes in behavior, excessive use of drugs, hallucinations, or hearing strange voices. Prolonged grief may cause uncomplicated bereavement where people feel remorseful about the death of their close ones, develop consistent thoughts about their death, feelings of worthlessness, display impaired psychomotor skills, and hallucinations unrelated to or in addition to a deceased individual.

Treatment

Mostly family and friends are the main support for the bereaved. Doctors, nurses, and therapists also play a significant role in helping mourners cope with their loss through grief counseling or grief therapy. Grief therapy is used when mourners display serious grief reactions. Some antidepressant medications help struggling patients with grief and depression (Ahmadimanesh et al., 2019).

Effects of Bereavement

It is true. Losing a loved one is life's most stressful event and can cause a high grade of destruction on physical and mental health (Smid et al., 2018). However, effects vary in severity, and for some people who already suffer from a mental health condition, they may be overwhelming.

Sleeping Difficulties

Bereavement disturbs regular sleep patterns, which is essential for the mind and body. As a result, people may wake up throughout the night or sleep too much. Winding down slowly before bed with something peaceful like taking a bath, reading a book, or performing breathing exercises may help people go to bed and wake up at the same time each day.

Fatigue

The roller-coaster of emotional trials drains the body's energy. Therefore, ensuring that one maintains a proper diet, exercising, and staying connected with family and friends are necessary tools to help one through grief.

Inflammation and Weakened Immune System

People experiencing grief may have a compromised ability to fight illness and infection. Talking to a mental health professional about your loss is a good idea. People may experience systematic inflammation, which occurs when the immune system responds to a threat. Bereavement can interfere with how the body responds to stress. People with comorbidities such as heart disease, arthritis, diabetes, asthma, and possibly cancer are at higher risk of experiencing more severe inflammation problems. Proper exercise and a proper diet can help to mitigate it.

Anxiety

A person with grief anxiety feels the change in thoughts and sensations, stomach cartwheels, increased heartbeat, or breathing rate. Talking to a mental health professional can be a good decision.

Depression

Numbness typically lasts a few hours to a few days, which indicates the beginning of depressive symptoms. In grief with depression, people often experience irritability and restlessness.

Statistics

Bereavement appears to increase the risk for mortality in the primary care database in the United Kingdom. According to a study by Perng & Renz (2018), older adults experience grief at a higher rate than younger adults or children, whereas spousal loss is common in older adults. Another data set shows that approximately 2.5 million people die annually in the United States, each leaving an average of five grieving people behind, and it is estimated that 1.5 million children lost one or both parents by age 15 (Cozza et al., 2017). Amerispeak and WebMD indicated that 57% of Americans are grieving the loss of their loved ones over the last three years (Zakarian et al., 2019).

The reviewed literature of Andrade (2018) indicates that about 7.2% of mourners experience the death of a parent or sibling, whereas one in every 14 American children experiences the death of a parent or sibling before age 18. The death of a parent (mother or father) has left approximately 1.5 million children living in a single-parent household (Dantchev et al., 2018). More than 70% of the elderly experience loss of a loved one over 30 months, as stated by Robbins-Welty et al. (2017).

Approximately 40% of mourners report depression symptoms one month after their loss, and 24% show signs after two months. However, over 7% of older men develop the mental health condition of Complicated Grief (CG). Up to 80% (Scocco et al., 2019) of men and women, after suicidal trial, seek professional help to handle the loss. Estimated prevalence rates for complicated grief among bereaved spouses range from 10% to 20% (LeRoy et al., 2020) due to elderly individuals following spousal loss. Moreover, Bartone et al. (2017) found bereaved elders experiencing less satisfaction and less hopefulness but a greater self-efficacy than those who were not bereaved. At the same time, undesirable social and health effects were significantly greater among women than men.

Conclusion

From this research, it appears that bereavement is one of the most severe, distressing, and traumatic events people experience in their life, but symptoms and responses to bereavement vary. Assessment of the challenges associated with bereavement is essential to understanding obstacles to bereaved individuals' adjustment while counseling and family or friend support to manage the loss. Though grief is not a disease, bereavement is associated with excess mortality risk, particularly in the early weeks and months after a loss. Additional research and clinical interventions are needed to target mourners at high risk of bereavement-related depression and stress disorders.

Research: Survival's Guilt

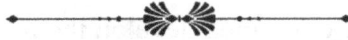

Survivors usually wonder why they lived while others lost their lives. Others believe that it was their fault that their loved ones died. Kettlyne could relate to the feeling of survival guilt because she felt that it was because of her hospitalization that her mother lost her life.

The concept of survivor guilt progressively appears in medicine, nursing, and psychology literature. Hutson et al. (2015) define survivor guilt as a perception related to the survivor's interpersonal process of surviving a life-threatening situation and harm while others died. Some feel guilty because they think they could have done more to save others' lives. Others feel guilty that another person died protecting them. The literature review of Valent (2016) indicates that survivor guilt is associated with an internal ethical decision aiming to modify instinctive survival strategies and preferences in a prosocial direction. However, emotional pain, shame, fairness are some ethical modifiers.

Survivor guilt was first debated and identified in veterans' survivors who survived Holocaust and 9/11 attacks. Survivors feel immense guilt after watching a loved one die, and for some reason, they survived. After decades, it has become clear that survivor's guilt is far more common than was first understood. Survivor's guilt is a symptom of PTSD, as stated in the recent version of the DSM-5. People demonstrate distorted feelings of guilt and negative thoughts about themselves. However, people can experience survivor's guilt without having PTSD and vice-versa.

Individuals who survive may productively modify their feelings of guilt into a sense of purpose. Moreover, they can also use survivor's guilt to cope with their feelings of helplessness and powerlessness in traumatic conditions. According to Murray (2018), survivor guilt signifies a connection with those who died because they believe that feelings of guilt keep the deceased's memories alive. This research will explore the concepts of survivor guilt and shame, explains why people go through survival guilt in the United States population, how it affects survivors' lives, and how it interferes with bereavement and the healing process after losing a loved one.

Conceptualization of Survivor Guilt and Shame

According to the findings of López-Castro et al. (2019), the concept of post-traumatic guilt and shame are significantly highlighted as a dimension of both complex and simple post-traumatic stress syndromes and received scant investigations in traumatology. The term "shame" is closely related to the emotions of survivor's guilt and is considered a self-conscious emotion. It occurs when people negatively judge themselves, whereas guilt occurs when people think of their actions and behavior unfavorably.

López-Castro et al. (2019) proposed critical and prolonged states of post-traumatic shame and guilt along with consequences across eight psycho-social dimensions, including:

- Self-attribution procedures

- Emotional states and capacity for regulatory effect

- Appraisal and interpretation of actions

- The impact of shame and guilt on personal identity

- Suicidality

- Defensive patterns

- Proneness to psychopathology (the scientific study of mental illness or disorders)

- PTSD

Felsen (2018) reported that survivors of the Holocaust experienced an intense feeling of guilt for living while others lost their lives. Early in the 1960s, psychoanalysts and psychiatrists from diverse areas in the United States defined survivor's guilt as survivor syndrome. Ruth Leys, the author of the book *From Guilt to Shame*, was the first to write about a genealogical-critical study of the vicissitudes of the concept of survivor guilt but the unrecognized implication of guilt's replacement by shame.

Effects of Survivor Guilt on Survivor's Life

People with survivor's guilt experience a severe impact on their daily life functions and face a high degree of fragmentation in their psychological and physical well-being. However, the degree and severity of a survivor's guilt vary from person to person. The most common psychological symptoms are:

- Feelings of helplessness,
- Flashbacks of the distressing incident
- Nightmares
- Irritability
- Anxiety
- mood swings
- Loss of motivation
- Aggressiveness
- Infatuated thoughts about the traumatic event and suicide
- Isolation

Similarly, common physical symptoms include loss of appetite or frequent appetite changes, difficulty sleeping, headache, nausea, stomachache, and heart palpitations.

Regret, Rumination, and Hindsight Bias

According to Watkins & Roberts (2020), people may experience regret and rumination over traumatic events. They may regret things they should have done to alter the outcome. Flashbacks of the incidents can further exacerbate feelings of guilt when individuals believe that their actions have worsened the consequences. In most cases of survivor's guilt, rumination is influenced by hindsight bias. People often tend to be biased by outcomes when viewing catastrophic events and overestimate their capability to have predicted the event's result to prevent the past occurrence. Hindsight bias distorts the memory. It becomes pervasive when survivors think about their missed chances and failures more deeply in judgment and regret that the circumstances could have turned out well if only a different choice had been made.

The experiment performed by Groß et al. (2017) revealed that participants experienced a higher degree of depressive symptoms focused on negative outcomes and completed more hindsight analyses. Though the relationship between depression and hindsight is accompanied by disappointment suggests a relationship to a malfunction of emotional regulation. However, individuals possessing a wide range of affect regulation strategies are flexible enough to adapt to stressful situations. During such times, guilt may have a legitimate cause, leading to another person's accident or death but little to no chance to prevent or change the results.

Causes of Survivor Guilt

Survivor's guilt is a syndrome that may occur in people who have experienced traumatic events such as natural catastrophes, accidents, terrorist acts, war or combat, rape, death threats, sexual violence, or severe injury. Survivor's guilt is a real syndrome that can seriously impact a person's life and cause debilitating side effects. People tend to internalize blame (as Kettlyne blamed herself for her mother's death, for example) and attribute connections to personal characteristics rather than external factors while explaining the events. Psychologists believe that people blaming themselves for events out of their control can be devastating. There is no absolute formula explaining the causes, but some experts have identified common factors that may intensify the risk of experiencing survivor's guilt.

History of Trauma

Research by Dye (2018) has indicated that people who experienced trauma during childhood can maximize the probability of negative emotions, life-threatening actions, and greater risk of causing survivor guilt. Moreover, continuous exposure to many traumatic events can increase guilt and shame and lead to severe symptoms.

Existing Mental Health Problems

According to DSM-5, people with a history of mental illness, particularly depression or anxiety, are more prone to experience survivor guilt and shame following trauma.

Contribution of Personality Factors

Usually, individuals struggling with low self-esteem may increase their self-criticism because they tend to reinforce their flaws and blame themselves as being incapable of doing anything right. Thus, they are exposed more frequently to a risk survivor's guilt than others.

No or Less Social Support

Evidence suggests that loneliness is detrimental to emotional health and can become even more overwhelming because people cannot share or express their feelings to others. In addition, a lack of social support means survivors might feel responsible for the incident and assume others blame them as well, fixating on false assumptions about the trauma. Research-based on the DSM-5 disorder criteria reveals that before and after trauma, societal support can help protect against the effects of PTSD.

Poor Coping Mechanism

Generally, people are more vulnerable to develop PTSD if they display avoidant styles of coping with distress. Avoidance coping includes cognitive and behavioral efforts that include social disengagement and wishful thinking (believing what one wishes to be true instead of the actual reality).

Use of Alcohol and Other Substances

It is impossible to suppress or evade traumatic memories to escape undesirable emotions, but people certainly try. In addition to social support, people get involved in drinking alcohol or substance abuse to numb emotional distress and find temporary relief. However, increased use of substances can worsen guilt and depression and may impose long-term adverse effects on their physical and mental well-being.

How Survivor Guilt Interferes with Bereavement and The Healing Process

Psychologists believe that there are always two parties involved in the death of a person: the one who dies and the bereaved survivors. The end of a loved one is always tragic and painful. It adversely affects survivors' lives and makes the healing process difficult for the bereaved after losing loved ones. The survivors react differently, depending upon the loss. For instance, sudden or unexpected death due to an accident, natural disaster, suicide or murder, significantly shakes the relational world's foundations. It challenges grief-stricken sufferers to find meaning in the loss and its aftermath.

However, the survivors' reactions may not be as intense following a death that occurs after a prolonged illness, and they may manage to cope with their grief after some time. Additional factors include lack of an opportunity to say goodbye, increased mourning phase duration, and the vulnerability of the bereaved toward survivor guilt.

A sudden death gives way to anticipatory grief when a loved one is diagnosed with a fatal disease. Coelho et al. (2018) say that anticipatory grief helps survivors prepare for upcoming loss and lessens the severity of the psychological reactions to the eventual death. When violent loss or death occurs, the mourners may experience frightening feelings ranging from fear to nervousness and powerlessness. Additionally, violent death provokes strong feelings of hostility in the griever, causing intense internal conflicts that lead to guilt, shame, and depression.

A different burden is faced by survivors with guilt, shame, and anger when a family member commits suicide. Individuals grieving such losses are commonly left with questions and blame themselves, wondering what they could or should have done to prevent the suicide. These questions remain unanswerable and may extend the procedure of grieving and coping with the loss. The natural and sudden loss of a loved one can be devastating and leave survivors with survivor syndrome. Survivors ask why they stayed safe while their loved one suffered and whether they did not try hard enough to prevent it.

Rational vs. Irrational Guilt

Some people feel guilty about actions they have carried out or took in the past. For instance, a drunk person may have hit someone while driving or killed an innocent in a gunshot incident. This type of guilt is known as rational guilt. Irrational guilt, in contrast, is related to actions over which they had no reasonable control, along with a feeling of what they should or should not have done to prevent the occurrence. Some tried to avoid the consequences but failed (Smith, 2020).

Prevalence of survivor guilt and Statistics in America

According to the results of a nationwide telephonic survey, approximately one-fourth of adults in the U.S. have experienced intense survivor guilt regardless of age, sex, and education. The incidence is strongly associated with depression (Luck & Luck-Sikorski, 2020). The prevalence of survivor guilt feelings with major depression was 37.4% compared to 8.1% in adults without depression. In other words, a considerable part of the adult population is confronted with survivor guilt feelings (Luck & Luck-Sikorski, 2020).

Coping with Survivor Guilt

In the findings of Stein et al. (2019), the guilt associated with surviving a life-threatening situation can be painful and challenging to overcome. Still, it is not impossible to cope with feelings of survivor guilt. A self-care routine is considered to be the most effective technique used for healing emotions of guilt. It comprises consistent physical movements, relaxing activities, a healthy diet, and sufficient rest. In addition, support from family and friends, sharing bad experiences, attending social support groups, advisors, and spiritual counselors are crucial components of coping with survivor guilt. A therapist may also contribute to helping individuals manage their painful emotions.

Conclusion

From this research, it appears that survivor syndrome widely describes the actions and responses of the people who have survived significant tragic events, such as the Holocaust. Holocaust survivors experienced various related symptoms, including anxiety and depression, intellectual impairment, social withdrawal, sleep disturbance and nightmares, physical complaints, and mood swings with loss of motivation. Several studies have examined the chronic nature of survivor's guilt that they have survived, and their family, friends, and colleagues did not. This condition, combined with a range of traumatic events, is now included under post-traumatic stress disorder in DSM-5. However, additional efforts must be taken to recognize situations under which feelings of guilt lead to adverse health-related outcomes and provide equivalent treatment approaches to cure this devastating health problem.

Chapter 5
Road to Recovery

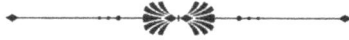

———— ···❦❦··· ————

Owning very few belongings, I moved into Sally's home in one trip. I transferred the home health care services, both physical therapy and wound care, to the new address. Within a month, despite still having orthopedic hardware in some places, my wounds had healed to where I could perform dressing changes on my own, and I was strong enough that I no longer required physical therapy in the home environment. Switching to outpatient rehab was uncomfortable but necessary. The facility visited had a lot of modern equipment, machines, and devices that were extremely helpful in restoring my balance and regaining my strength.

No longer qualifying for transportation services, I had to rely on friends and family to go to the rehab location. Arriving late meant I missed the window of opportunity to undergo therapy and would be rescheduled for another day. Lacking reliable transportation, I missed quite a few appointments. Plagued with therapy inconsistencies, I failed to improve to the point where I began to lose strength and mobility. To improve the chances of making a better recovery, with the help of my husband, I borrowed an old but functioning vehicle and began to drive.

I had not sat in the driver's seat since the day of my accident. The casts and hardware on my legs were located at my ankles and limited my ability to move freely. I used my right foot to accelerate and my left foot to brake. As difficult as that was, physical debility was the least of my worries. After chauffeuring myself around the block a few times, without warning, a sudden rush of emotional memories caused my heart rate and breathing to race. It felt like I had been pulled from the present and dropped into the past in an upside-down car on Interstate 95. I had to pull over, breathe deeply and try to shake off the awful fear causing me distress. I had to make a conscious effort to stop thinking about the accident on my twenty-fourth birthday.

Despite my progress at the rehab using the walker, there was difficulty and slowness in initiating walking, which eased once I generated a little momentum. Transitioning to a cane took a long time, approximately a year and a half. The orthopedic hardware and the surgeries did their job, but my ankles had become fused, and the joints developed arthritis. As a result of the arthritis, the rehab discharged me from therapy.

The orthopedic physician advised me that I was permanently disabled, and ankle fusion reversal would be necessary to improve the chances of recovery. Another operation was the last thing I needed to hear. There would be a three-month period of convalescence before being able to receive physical therapy and bear weight. After my mother's death, I no longer had the support system that I originally had. There was no way I was going to agree to further debility now that I was able to walk.

I needed to go back to work. I had no income, and living off Sally was unfair. A few months earlier, while at the trauma center, a social worker helped me apply for Medicaid. After discharge, I received food stamps. However, I was denied cash assistance because I was legally married. The fact that my husband was not at all supportive did not matter. Being married worked against me as it limited my receiving help.

I had my son and brother to take care of. Desperate to earn some income while considering the limitations of my current vulnerabilities, I began to explore my options. Trying to return to the ambulance or hospital position was out of the question. Instead, I needed a job that I could do from behind a desk. With the help of the Internet, I applied to several office positions. One interview was for a customer service position at a telephone company.

The human resources representative was surprised to receive a job applicant saddled in a wheelchair and sporting bilateral lower extremity casts and orthopedic boots. Before my appearance became an issue, I explained that I needed the job to feed my dependents. Luckily, I was hired. I had not worked for a very long time, and being employed again gave me a sense of independence.

A mere few days into my new job, I realized how harmful the activity was to my recovery process. By noon, my legs would swell, and the pain was unbearable. I could not take pain medication while at work because it made me drowsy, and I could not drive home impaired. The only alternative was to endure the pain throughout the entire shift. Each day was a new struggle. Finally, the challenges started to pile up, and I had to resign after a few weeks of holding on. Unfortunately, my eagerness to get back to work ended up delaying the healing progress. Four long months of convalescence were necessary before I would work again.

At home, I put myself through an exercise regimen. It was not too strenuous, and I got plenty of rest. When I felt ready, free from the confines of a wheelchair but still using a cane as an assistive device, I reached out to my former manager at the hospital. She was leery of hiring me because of my physical limitations. I understood her concerns and waited a few days for a decision. When the call never came, I contacted her boss, the department director.

My timing could not have been better. The director was getting ready to retire. She was aware of my hospitalization and all the other difficulties I had experienced. This woman took it upon herself to help me as much as she could. She created a secretarial position to accommodate me because she knew that I could not stand on my feet for too long. The manager was not too happy because I had gone over her head, and a position had been created just for me. She took it personally. I regretted taking that step, but I was in dire need.

To my surprise, my old co-workers were not all thrilled to have me back. I thought I would be embraced by everyone. Antagonism and indifference were not the responses I expected from men and women who had been so supportive during my hospitalization. Although some staff members were helpful and understanding, the head secretary and head nurse intentionally sabotaged me. I wish I were exaggerating.

One of the tasks I was instructed to consistently perform was going to the mailroom located in the hospital's basement to retrieve envelopes and packages. It was a long and strenuous walk that took me an hour to complete. Upon my return, they asked why such a simple task was taking so long. Both women knew perfectly well that I had just started to walk again and still had limitations. As much as I tried to conceal my discomfort, slow movements and cautious sitting and standing gave away that I had not completely healed. Whenever the opportunity arose, one or the other would mention that I was not fit to do the work I had been assigned. I was asked to consider resigning for the sake of my continued health and wellbeing. When that did not work, they would nitpick at the most unimportant details of my work. I remained respectful and courteous in a sea of uneasy relationships where being hypercritical was the norm. Up until then, I had not thought it possible that adults could be bullied.

Quitting was not going to happen. I was responsible for the care of a very young child and a teenager who was not yet ready to begin working. Instead of giving up, I put my nose to the grindstone, dove deep into my duties, and kept a smile on my face while I kept plugging away. It was important to maintain the façade of emotional and physical energy and pretend that no task was too demanding. Once I got to my car, my sanctuary, feeling wronged and mistreated, I would burst into tears on the drive home. After every shift, without fail, my feet would get so badly swollen that Sally had to help me remove my shoes.

One evening as I was heading to work, I was stopped by a police officer. I was not speeding. I did not recall rolling past a stop sign. I had no clue what I did wrong. I was instructed to turn off the engine and step out of the vehicle with my license and registration when I attempted to ask. As I attempted to reach into the back seat to grab my cane, the police officer snapped into a defensive position, drew his firearm, and shouted, "Hands up, now!"

I did as the officer instructed and began trembling and crying. There were more commands, but I did not hear his words with a gun pointed at me. I dropped my head as if not looking at him would somehow deescalate the situation and raised my arms higher to signify complete submission. It may have helped.

When I regained my composure, in a stern tone, I stammered, "I'm disabled! I was just reaching for my cane!"

Imagine getting shot over a cane. Had I survived, there would have been many more months of hospitalization.

After confirming my contention, the weapon was holstered, and the police officer apologized. He knelt next to my door and sincerely apologized, explaining that his job is inherently dangerous, and it had been scary for him working nights.

I told him I was glad he was not trigger-happy because I would have died. Then, with a sly smile, he told me I had nothing to fear because he knew CPR. And with good-humored bantering, the nightmare was over as quick as it had begun. The reason for asking me to step out was to look at a flickering taillight. He wanted me to open the trunk so that he could remove the bulb for me.

Continuing toward work, I was distraught thinking about the muzzle of that gun pointed at me. Had it gone wrong, the newspaper headline would read, "Woman fatally shot by police during a traffic stop for brandishing a cane."

I understand the officer's reaction. Any reasonable person in the same position would have feared for his life. Nonetheless, it was traumatizing. The incident sapped the strength and weakening the resolve that I was saving for another long night at work.

At work, as I shared the tale with a few trusted colleagues, I cried out, "Oh my goodness, this cane is going to be the death of me one day!"

One of my co-workers remarked that the cane might be cursed. Everyone laughed, including me. He asked for a closer look, and I handed it to him.

Looking me in the eye, he took a few steps back and insisted that I stand up and take the cane from his hand. Was he serious? I depended on the cane to walk. I needed that cane.

I cried out, "Do you think that if I could walk without it, I would still be using it?"

"Just try," he insisted. "We are all here. We won't let you fall."

My legs felt strong. I decided to take on the challenge. I stood, steadied myself, and took a small, successful step. Then another and another. All the while, my focus was on my feet.

"Hey," he smugly beamed, "look at how far you got."

I had not noticed he kept backing away as I shambled toward him. I could not believe I had walked across the length of the nursing station without the cane. The possibility of overexerting myself, twisting a joint, or experiencing a fall did not frighten me.

Overjoyed and inappropriately using my outdoor voice, I proclaimed, "I can walk without that thing!"

The co-worker who encouraged me raised his arms high and declared, "Mission accomplished!"

He was not teasing me as I had originally suspected. His goal was to help build up my self-confidence. It proved to be an unexpected and incredibly emotional moment for me. It felt like a Super Bowl victory, and I celebrated it by sharing a group embrace with everyone. From that eye-opening moment forward, I felt more empowered. I was not aware that I had built up the strength to walk without assistive devices.

Uncertainty was a thing of the past. With confidence soaring, I was able to translate the new conviction not only into the work that I was doing but it also inspired me to join a gym. Thanks to all the physical therapists who had helped me in the past, I had a fair idea of the exercises that I needed to practice. Throughout the long months of workouts that followed, I managed to shed some of the extra weight that I had put on during the recovery process. It was not easy, not in the slightest. I experienced occasional setbacks; my legs would sometimes swell, and the pain prevented me from pushing forward, but only temporarily because resilience and perseverance were my two allies. Surrendering was not a word in my vocabulary.

Walking is something people take for granted until the ability is lost. However, I learned that it is not as easy as putting one foot in front of the other. Learning to walk again in the wake of physical and emotional debility requires a deliberate and purposeful commitment. It would have been easy to give up and return to using assistive devices or even continue to waddle as I had done when I first became free of the cane.

Thanks to a positive attitude and the willingness to complete tasks at work, I had slowly but surely won over most of the staff. I thought about asking for their help regarding one more thing: I needed their support evaluating my walking and correcting me when I failed to ambulate correctly. My initial concern was that my request could be interpreted as an ongoing weakness, but, in fact, appealing for help demonstrated my desire to get better. It was a show of strength rather than weakness. Therefore, I recruited a few of my colleagues to be my accountability partners. These people would monitor my walking and keep me on track toward the goal of walking normally once more. I asked them to stop me any time they noticed I was doing the duck wobble. They understood that bringing me a wheelchair or handing me a cane were not solutions. These incredible people, professionals in many different healthcare fields, kept me going. I was fortunate to have them by my side.

Research: Social Rejection

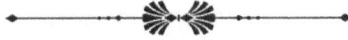

———————— ❧❧ ————————

Kettlyne was on her road to recovery yet experienced a degree of social rejection. One would have thought that everyone would have welcomed her back with open arms because of the great obstacles that she had to overcome to get on the road to recovery. To belong and be accepted is a fundamental need of every human being. Our ancestors survived the harsh environments by depending on small groups of people. Ever since, belongingness has become a mode of survival. Though we do not have to face the same harsh environment as our ancestors, there is now an ever-growing need to feel accepted and belong due to different but even more severe kinds of survival. When this need is satisfied, it becomes the cause for good mental and emotional health. On the contrary, when this need is not satisfied, it causes perceived or actual social rejection. In this paper, we attempt to discuss the crucial role of social rejection in people's lives and its severe consequences.

Definition of Social Rejection

Social rejection can be defined as a deliberate exclusion of an individual from social relationships or social interaction. The rejection may be interpersonal (family) or by peers, or it could be romantic rejection. The rejection could be by a whole group or by an individual. Social rejection might be passive in the form of "silent treatment," or it could also be active in the form of daily bullying, teasing, or aggression. Social rejection is a subjective concept. The individual perceives it through their own personal lens, and consequently, the rejection could be sometimes perceived rather than actual. In either case, the consequences on mental health are the same.

The Impact of Being Rejected

Social rejection is something that every human being tries to avoid in their lives, and although it is somehow inevitable, some people are more sensitive to such rejection compared to others. The people who are more vulnerable and constantly perceive rejection and exclusion have been found in research studies to have lower self-esteem than those who perceive themselves to be accepted by others. When people believe that they are not accepted and not included by others, a range of emotions arises in the human brain. Seven emotions are observed to be involved when people perceive that their relational value to other people is low or in potential jeopardy, including hurt feelings, jealousy, loneliness, shame, guilt, social anxiety, and embarrassment (Leary, 2015).

The Pain of Social Rejection

Hurt feelings have been called a "rejection emotion" due to two important reasons. One being the obvious emotional hurt an individual feels when they realize they do not have the same position in someone's life as they have always perceived. The second is that neurological studies have revealed that the human brain shows the same response to social rejection as being physically hurt. As far as the brain is concerned, a broken heart may not be so different from a broken arm.

The cyber ball technique is commonly used to test this phenomenon under functional magnetic resonance imaging (fMRI). The subject plays an online game of catch with two other players, and the other players eventually exclude that person from the game, playing catch only with each other. The subject's brain shows increased activity in the dorsal anterior cingulate and the anterior insula, the two regions that normally show activity in response to physical pain.

Interpersonal Rejection

Rejection, no matter the source, affects the individual without a doubt. However, rejection from close relations (family, friends, and romantic partners) definitely has more profound effects than rejection from strangers. It just hurts more and has a more significant impact. Rejection from those who are an essential part of our lives can be one of the most distressing and consequential events. (See how Kettlyne felt when her husband turned away from her during her healing process.) Whether the rejection consists of complete outcast or just casual ignorance, it profoundly affects the emotional and psychological state. In fact, human behavior is greatly influenced by the desire to avoid rejection. Interpersonal rejection causes an immediate negative emotional response in the individual (mostly low self-esteem) followed by motivated behavior, which can either be pro-social, anti-social, or withdrawal/avoidance.

Repeated Rejections and Burnout

If these interpersonal rejections continue, it can lead to a person losing their confidence and listing these repeated rejections as personal failures. Repeated rejections cause an individual to become cynical and unmotivated and often lead to burnout. Burnout is a state of persistent stress that generates physical and emotional tiredness and eventually a lack of interest (Jaremka et al., 2020). Burnout usually occurs from feeling overwhelmed. It makes you question your self-worth and the value of your hard work. People who are constantly rejected by their loved ones can experience burnout when they are left to feel that their efforts are not enough to sustain the relationship.

Burnout includes feelings such as:

- Helplessness
- Feeling unappreciated

- Exhausted

- Unmotivated

- Losing interest

- Feeling that you've reached your upper limit

- Feeling overwhelmed

- Close to quitting

- Not caring about a relationship anymore.

Consequences of Social Rejection

Social rejection can have long-term consequences. Repeated rejection is often internalized by individuals, leaving them with severe emotional and psychological dysfunctions. These severe consequences can easily hinder progress in life.

Trauma

Social rejection can leave a person traumatized. For example, children who face rejection from parents in early life become traumatized and struggle to succeed academically, and struggle to make and maintain relationships later in life.

Low Self-Esteem

Rejection lowers self-esteem and instills a constant fear of rejection in the individual. That constant fear holds the person back from taking opportunities, whether regarding career choices or entering relationships. The person's fear of not getting accepted hinders him/her from trying anything in life.

Depression

Social rejection in its active form, which is bullying, is the leading cause of depression and self-harm in teens. Other than bullying, causes of depression may include a lack of support in times of need and facing the avoidance of loved ones.

Mental Conditions

Social rejection can exasperate already present mental conditions, such as stress and anxiety. In addition, rejection overwhelms the individual, which can worsen the anxiety responses. The constant fear of rejection will also put more stress and anxiety and aggravate the symptoms.

Aggression

The feeling that a person is devalued in the family or even elsewhere may cause anger and lead to aggressive behavior. For example, multiple domestic abuse incidents, school shootings, and lashing out at a romantic partner, all instigated by social rejection. These kinds of outbursts damage relationships and careers almost permanently.

Coping with Social Rejection

Dealing with social rejection depends largely on dealing and coping with the negative feelings that arise as a reaction to social rejection. The goal should be to minimize internal pain.

Be Mindful of Your Self-Esteem

It is essential to remember your self-worth and not let rejections damage it. This can be a difficult thing to practice, but one's self-esteem can be protected with effort. One thing that might help is to understand others' perspectives and not let their decisions define the worth of oneself.

Beware of Disrupted Cognitive Patterns

Sometimes individuals develop disrupted thought patterns due to previous bad experiences or schemas. As a result, they overgeneralize and personalize situations and other people's reactions. By looking out for these patterns in your own thoughts, a person can cope with and understand such situations more effectively.

Self-Care and Self-Improvement

In the event of social rejection, one thing that can help cope is focusing on the good things about oneself. For example, bringing attention to what makes you feel good rather than an opinion of someone else can help a person cope better. Also, channeling one's energy into improving oneself instead of stressing is a healthy coping mechanism.

Take Time to Process

If a person is dealing with repeated rejections, it is essential to take time and process each rejection separately and not become overwhelmed. Take time before reaching out for another opportunity, and only reach out when you are ready again. The constant struggle only leads to overwhelming feelings and burnout. It is crucial to take a break and be easy on yourself. Take time to digest the events and move forward only when ready.

Seek help from Colleague, Mentor, or Professional

There is no reason for an individual to deal with rejection alone. Although social rejection may make an individual feel like he/she is isolated and it becomes harder to trust others, there is always someone a person can reach out to and talk to. If there is no one in your personal circle, you can always reach out to a professional for help.

Be Persistent and Look Out for Opportunities

Giving up on oneself is usually what makes a person feel depressed and helpless. Thinking that social acceptance defines their self-worth and that one rejection equals the ultimate end gives birth to a fear of never being accepted and thus never trying again. Being persistent and continually looking for new opportunities will make the person realize that there are so many more places in this world where they can belong, and they do not need to stop with one rejection.

Conclusion

The scope and scale of emotions that arise from social rejection point towards how vital interpersonal relations are to our mental health and the need to belong and be accepted by others are to human beings. Human beings are inherently motivated to be valued by others and especially by those close to them. Yet every now and then, people have to face minor or major rejections in life. Therefore, it is crucial to find ways of coping in such events and, just as importantly, to support others looking for a place to belong.

Chapter 6
I Didn't Sign Up for This

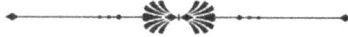

———— ❧❧ ————

Marriage is a celebration, a ceremony, a commitment, a union. Two people declare their love by standing before family and friends and exchange vows and rings. In sickness and in health, they will journey through life together, no longer lonely. For richer or poorer, no matter how challenging that may be, professing love for one another is intended to be lasting until death. As it turned out, that was not the script intended for my life.

When I was involved in a life-altering automobile accident in 2001, my husband was the most supportive person in my life, always at my side, visiting me at all hours of the day, making me feel safe when surgeons were doing what they could to save my limbs. He had been there for the good times and now for the bad. But, as time went by and healing failed to progress to his satisfaction, my husband began to visit with less frequency. I noticed how the concern for my wellbeing faded from his heart. It disappeared simultaneously with the twinkle of love I used to see in his eyes. He could not hide the look of disappointment and disgust. All he saw was a deformed woman lying on a hospital bed, nothing more. Who wouldn't be discouraged? Of course, there would be a strain on the marriage!

I knew the situation was difficult for him. It would be difficult for anyone. I made excuses for his absence. I figured, if I could not look at my own deformities, how could he bear it? I was no longer the woman wearing a white dress and long train with whom he walked down the aisle. That young woman had vanished into the ether, and there was no guarantee she would ever be able to find her way back to good health. I should not have been surprised that my husband decided to abandon the marriage within the first few weeks of my debility. He did not even try to maintain appearances throughout the most critical period of my distress.

Even with creative embellishments, wedding vows take a few brief minutes to verbalize. Two souls become one as the cherished moment is immortalized in photographs and video forever. The journey can be everlasting with trust, respect, compassion, honesty, and other virtues, but no one knows what the future holds in store for a blissful couple. Standing at the altar, at a magical place and an enchanted time, caught up in the fairytale dream, it is easy to believe a couple will share a kiss and live happily ever after. But, of course, it is impossible to gauge the depth of meaning that each person is expressing even at this advanced stage of a relationship.

Some people may enter matrimony with thoughts of fraud and deception. I do not believe this was the case with my husband. We had been together since junior high school. Our marriage represented young love blossoming into a mature, lifelong romance and commitment. We had always done everything together – I used to think of him as my best friend forever (BFF)! However, when one thing went wrong and then another, the dominoes started crashing down around me. When a marriage slips into trouble, the cause can be finances, disease, addiction, infidelity, poor communication, or any number of hardships. At the age of twenty-four, fate delivered onto me many difficult moments. With the power to choose a direction, I decided to get better and try my best to return to happy family life. Unfortunately, my husband did not have the faith or patience to choose a positive path. He turned his back on his wife and son and chose a selfish and harmful route to follow. My Romeo was gone. My relationship was dead. And while at many different points of I felt weakened by one bad experience after another, I never gave up because I had a son who needed me.

After a long journey through rehab, self-motivated exercise, and a lot of physical and emotional pain, I was able to get back on my feet and move out of Sally's house. I maintained my employment and had earned enough income to rent my own place. I made progress. Yet, things with my husband deteriorated to the point where he had not bothered to call his own son for months. He only visited his wife and son one time since I was released from the hospital.

One day, when I worked up the courage to find out what was keeping him so busy, with very little effort, I discovered he was having a relationship with a girl we both knew from high school.

The betrayal was heartbreaking. How could he do this to me? I knew things were bad, but where was the loyalty? He made a promise, and I expected nothing less. Neither of us signed up to lose a home due to arson. I certainly did not plan on disabling myself in a car wreck, but infidelity? That was not okay.

I am ashamed and embarrassed to admit that I still hoped that my husband would return once I could explain that I was much better. I could not bring myself to push him away and shut him out. That is, I hung onto a positive frame of mind until the day he told me he could not deal with a crippled wife. He shared a litany of poor excuses and harsh criticisms that made me doubt the relationship we once shared and, worst of all, made me give up on him. My optimism sank to the lowest depths of the darkest well. The icing on top of the cake was when he put the new woman in his life before our son.

I could accept that it would no longer be husband, wife, and child, but husband and mistress with a son that did not matter was a bitter pill to swallow. My son and I were no longer considered relevant in his life. This man went as far as tattooing the image of his girlfriend on his body. I felt disrespected. It was as if commitment meant nothing to him. The nerve of this man. What was he thinking?

I am a firm believer in not being judgmental, but it is difficult to respect a woman dating a married man. Perhaps the relationship would have been easier to accept had my husband begun dating after divorcing me. It beats becoming a liar and a cheat and putting one's family through agony. To make matters worse, perhaps because there was nothing else to talk about, my husband shared a relatively large amount of family secrets with his girlfriend, things such as relatives with illnesses, poor investments, failed businesses, etc. He needlessly made both of us vulnerable by pouring his heart out to this woman.

Whenever I tried to speak to my husband regarding our son, insurance, or other important issues, the conversation somehow went south, and the mudslinging would begin. I heard the girlfriend say I could not do anything for him because I was crippled and that she was a better partner because she was not impaired. The abusive nature of this type of behavior is meant to destroy the victim's resolve. As upset as I wanted to be at his girlfriend, I knew that it had only gotten to this level because my husband had made it possible.

Whenever parents bicker and shout, it is always the children who pay the price, whatever the reason. Although parental responsibility should not end when a matrimonial relationship leads to separation or divorce, it sometimes does when one parent chooses to walk away from the child. Knowing that any contact would lead to a verbal dispute, I tried to limit my interaction with my husband to when our son was asleep, and I made every imaginable effort to keep a civil tone so that I would not wake him.

I have no doubt that my husband and his partner in crime were intentionally using my son as a weapon to hurt me. This bitter and vengeful conduct negatively impacted an innocent child who in no way deserved their indirect contempt. It was heart-wrenching to see my little boy sitting by the window, wondering when his father would visit. Both my husband and his girlfriend should have been ashamed of themselves. Instead of being mature and responsible, he never changed his ways and continued to disappoint our son. The conflict between us only escalated as time went by. The girlfriend became more prominent in his life, she was his shield of protection, and I had to go through her to speak to him.

One distressful incident occurred between my husband and me that still wakes me in horror to this day. Without warning, without requesting permission, my husband picked up our son from school and disappeared without a trace. I did not discover he had snatched our son away until I arrived at the school. It was an unexpected and frightening occurrence that is still difficult to think about to this day. His blatant disregard for my feelings was unforgivable.

I called the police and accused my husband of kidnapping. Unfortunately, since we were still legally married and there was no court order defining physical custody, the father had the right to take the child. Since there was no crime, the police could not help me find my son.

For the next two weeks, I wore out my fingers dialing phone numbers attempting to reach my husband and anyone who knew him. All calls to his number went straight to voicemail, he never responded. My brother and I scoured the city and visited all his old haunts. No one had seen him. Not even his family knew his whereabouts. At least that is what they told me. I could not eat, I could not sleep, I could not focus at work.

I had no idea how my child was doing. He was only four years old. Was he being fed? Was he being taken care of? Was the girlfriend abusing him in any way? I could not control racing thoughts of my son wandering through the streets and being killed. I was so afraid of the situation escalating into a scenario where my little boy would lose his life. I was very angry, outraged, as any mother would be.

Fourteen days after taking our son out of school, the school notified me that my husband dropped him off without a word of explanation. With my heart pounding and fluttering, I raced to the school to pick up my son. The anguish and insanity had finally come to an end. I was relieved and happy, but more importantly, I had worked up the courage and conviction to end the toxic situation that was causing harm.

The number one priority was to transfer my son to a new school so that this nightmare could not happen again. The second order of business was to move to a gated community with restricted access. The next step was to contact an attorney and file for divorce, an action that I had resisted up until then because I wanted to repair the relationship.

Until the kidnapping episode, a dissolution of marriage was not something I had considered because we had been a couple since we were teenagers. The first boy I kissed, my first boyfriend, my husband, he was my first everything. By the age of nineteen, we were married with a baby on the way. We began adult, independent lives at a young age, and I thought we would grow old together as we promised one another on our wedding day. However, the recent emotional wounds were too deep, and flushing the ten-year relationship was no longer difficult. All hesitation and reluctance were gone.

The attorney I hired was the right person for the job. He was an experienced professional who tried his best to make the process orderly and efficient. Since my husband, the defendant, had abandoned his familial duties, I thought the legal action would be easier, less involved, and less stressful than it turned out to be.

However, my husband's games continued. He tried to prolong the divorce process by intentionally not showing up for court. The man went as far as quitting his job to avoid the financial responsibility he owed to his son. To his detriment, there is no hiding from the divorce action, and he soon exhausted every sly trick he could think of to avoid the court-ordered child support agreement.

I was not interested in pursuing the matter any further. It was now up to me as a single mother to shoulder the financial needs of my son. However, my ex-husband had one final trick up his sleeve. After all the hassles, after walking out on his hospitalized wife, after the infidelity, after the emotional torture, after kidnapping our son, and after toying with the court, the man expressed he wanted to reconcile and save the marriage. This last, desperate act revealed his opportunistic personality.

The extramarital affair he had initiated had ended, and he realized that the grass was not greener on the other side. The only thing he could do was try to worm his way back into my heart. Too bad for him. There was no going back for me. Knowing what I went through, knowing he could do it again, the man had no place in my life. I was done with him.

My journey of personal growth began with a series of monumental setbacks, all within one year. Every step I took forward was met with two steps back. I was not strong, I gave up many times, but I was fortunate enough to meet the right people to help me along the way. Sometimes it was a friend, and sometimes a stranger, who pointed the way and helped me focus on the path toward physical and emotional recovery. Thanks to these relationships, thanks to people who shared a word of wisdom, encouragement, and hope, I was able to find the strength to conquer doubt and fear and make better decisions that served to propel me to the next breakthrough and the next and the next. It is important to know that the Almighty God knows when to present a person with the right words of inspiration at the right moment in their lives. Sometimes the words can be disguised, easily dismissed, or outright ignored. But, afterward, the hidden message and meaning will take shape. I learned that it was always possible to create a positive ripple in the most negative situation, whatever the situation.

Thinking about all the things I had lost was an anchor dragging me to the depths of despair. I often asked the Lord how much more he would put in my path, how much more was required of me. In my prayers, as I wept, I told God I could not handle any more loss, any more debility, any more pain. I soon learned that hardship is an inevitable part of life, and hardship has meaning as unpleasant and unwelcome as it is. It has a purpose. Everything happens for a reason, and God is in control of all things. If you lose a job, there is a better job coming. If your husband leaves you, a better husband is coming.

I grew up in the church, and I have always known that God will never give you more than you can handle. When we are being tested by the Lord, it may not occur that the obstacles in our path are not beyond our abilities to withstand and overcome challenges. When we are confronted with adversity, we must remember to keep pushing forward. When we are enduring troubles, we must remember that the struggle is not going to last forever. There is light at the end of every tunnel. This is a life code to live by.

Research: Low Self-Esteem

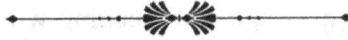

By now, there was a lot that happened to Kettlyne, trauma after trauma chipping away at her mental well-being, confidence, and sense of self-worth; it is no wonder that her self-esteem was so severely impacted. Kettlyne's low self-esteem resulted from a lot of things happening one after the other, but it can happen to anyone. Self-love is vital to our beings. If you think about the things you hate and the things you love, you will realize how indifferent we are about ourselves. Thus, we see the constant self-indulgence and need for attention. Self-esteem is a crucial construct in clinical, developmental, personality, and social psychology. Its role in psychological functioning has been studied for nearly a century (Greenier, Kernis, and Waschull, as cited in Abdel-Khalek, 2016). Over the past 35 years, more than 18,000 studies exploring self-esteem have been published. It is, therefore, safe to say that the research on self-esteem is of such gravity and scope that it is almost impossible to summarize, yet we can extract some vital points regarding the subject.

Definition of Self-Esteem

Self-esteem is usually presented as a continuum, with the lowest and highest are extremes and the middle are appropriate. Commonly used, self-esteem is a favorable view of oneself. In his first publication in 1980, *Principles of Psychology*, William James defined self-esteem as "success divided by pretensions." This concept paints an intriguing perspective regarding self-esteem. The idea is that it can be promoted by achieving greater successes and maintained by avoiding failures. But there is a gray area, as it can also be increased by adopting less ambitious goals: "to give up pretensions is as blessed a relief as to get them gratified" (James, 1890, p. 311).

On the other hand, a simpler concept of self-esteem is defined as an individual's overall positive self-evaluation. High self-esteem consists of respecting himself and considering himself worthy (Rosenberg, as cited in Abdel-Khalek, 2016). Wang and Ollendick (2001) define self-esteem as an evaluation of oneself followed by an emotional reaction towards oneself.

Belongingness

The sense of belonging or feeling accepted, liked, and included by others, is a primary need of human beings. It is human nature to crave a sense of belonging. Abraham Maslow (1970) was the first to identify "belongingness" as a basic human need; in his *Hierarchy of Needs,* he ranked it right after the need for safety. Studies have proved that self-esteem and self-worth have an empirical link with perceived or actual belongingness. After an extensive review of the empirical literature, Baumeister and Leary (1995) found evidence that pathological consequences of a medical, psychological, and behavioral nature are more likely when belonging needs are not met.

Effects of Low Self-Esteem

People with low self-esteem suffer from feelings of worthlessness, inferiority, and emotional instability, leading to dissatisfaction with life. Research has shown that lower self-esteem has a gigantic role in many behavioral and emotional dysfunctions. Compared to people with high self-esteem, people with lower self-esteem tend to be more shy, unhappy, jealous, anxious, depressed, and lonely. They are also more likely to jeopardize their health and others, such that they are more prone to dangers, including teenage pregnancy, criminal behavior, aggression, and substance abuse. [11]

Self-Esteem and Psychopathology

Lower self-esteem has also been shown to be a trigger of many mental health conditions. For example, low self-esteem combined with stressful events elevates and triggers depressive symptoms. In addition, according to *Anxiety-Buffer Hypothesis,* self-esteem acts as a shield (buffer) against mental health threats – fear and loneliness – thus hampering anxiety and depressive symptoms. When a crisis happens, people with lower self-esteem do not have the resources to cope with that crisis and thus are more likely to spiral down into depression or anxiety.

Lower Self-Esteem and Destructive Behavioral Patterns

A study by Andreassen, Pallesen, and Griffiths (2016) showed a negative correlation between self-esteem and internet addiction, illustrating how it is used as a means to inhibit negative self-evaluation. Lower self-esteem has also been related to alcohol and substance abuse, maladaptive perfectionism, and suicidal tendencies. As Daniel Katz, an American psychologist, said, "If there were ever a magic bullet that could transform a young person's life, it would be a pill coated with self-esteem. This powerful yet fragile quality is the key to the future for a teenager."

Importance of Self-Esteem

Having lower or higher self-esteem dictates what decisions a person makes in his/her life. People with higher self-esteem make choices towards success. They are more motivated and open to exploring new things, whereas people with low self-esteem focus more on their failures. People who have high self-esteem are more likely to take care of themselves and be more optimistic. In addition, they have more intimate and genuine relationships with friends and family.

Conversely, people with low self-esteem believe that they are not worthy of care and happy outcomes or often think that they are not capable of achieving them, so they let the good things slip. They are also less resilient in dealing with adversaries because they underestimate their skills and capabilities. Lower self-esteem makes a person more vulnerable to mental health illnesses and other severe behavioral and emotional issues. In contrast, having good self-esteem makes people healthy mentally and emotionally. It provides a healthy coping source to fight stressful situations and maintain an inner balance.

Sources of Self-Esteem

To find out what causes low self-esteem, it is important to first find the roots of self-esteem. This way, we can better understand what's negatively impacting it and bolster it when possible. Research on the sources of self-esteem has revealed results quite the opposite to what was expected, and it has made the researchers reconsider some of their previous preconceptions.

We can divide these sources into three categories (Emler, 2001, pp. 35-42):

1. Factors having minimum or no effect
2. Factors having moderate effect
3. Factors having significant effect

Factors having Minimum or No Effect

Factors that were suspected to affect self-esteem but were found to have little or no effect include ethnicity, race, social class, and gender. For example, studies among black and White people groups found no considerable differences in their self-esteem; on the contrary, Black people were found to have generally higher self-esteem than White people. The reason could be that people's self-esteem depends on the approval of their own close friends and family rather than the approval of strangers in society (Gray-Little, Hafdahl, as cited in Emler, 2001).

When it comes to social class, it only affects the adults mildly. It does not affect adolescents or children because it has nothing to do with their personal capability. Instead, it is something they have inherited, whereas, for adults, it is a challenge to their capabilities and skills to change that status quo.

Kling et al. (1999) explored 216 studies of gender differences in self-esteem. The results revealed that globally men have higher self-esteem than women; the differences were consistent but small. These differences are often attributed to the general differences between the two genders, that is, the basic features that are required for certain gender to achieve (for example, men are supposed to be masculine and tough). These circumstances can disproportionately damage the self-esteem of both genders.

Factors having a Moderate Effect

Elements found to have a modest effect on self-esteem include successes and failures, rejection and acceptance, and appearance. The general expectation is that successes are supposed to increase self-esteem, and failures are supposed to weaken it. Still, experiments found that the impact of success and failure on self-esteem is rather temporary. Part of the reason could be that there are other options for explaining performance that has few implications for one's worth as a person – for example, it could be bad luck, less effort, or less time. The point is that success and failure only affect a person's self-esteem up to a certain point.

Researchers used the data from the U.S. *National Longitudinal Study of Youth,* which contains details regarding young people's self-esteem during high school and information about their after-education employment. They were successful in determining that lower self-esteem was related to unemployment and unsatisfactory employment. However, it is also important to note that these experiences that represent acceptance or rejection are differences in self-esteem rather than the direct source.

When it comes to appearance, the basic assumption should be that physical appearance should correlate with self-esteem. With all the beauty standards and the desire to be attractive, self-esteem is supposed to be compromised by a person's appearance. But here is a fact about self-esteem: it is dependent on self-evaluation, not reality. So basically, appearance affects self-esteem depending on what a person believes about his/her appearance and not the opinion of uninvolved observers (excluding friends and family members).

Factors having a Significant Effect

The most substantial factor found to affect self-esteem is parents and their behavior. The researchers explained this common notion in how our own image of ourselves impacts self-esteem more than what others think of us. Still, in the case of parents, they too realize that it is hard not to accept their perspective and opinion when we are living with them. Thus, the first contribution regarding the vital role of parents in self-esteem provided four behavioral qualities that impact the children's self-esteem (Coopersmith, as cited in Emler, 2001):

- The amount of acceptance, approval, and affection shown

- The extent to which clear standards of behavior were promoted and expected

- The degree to which discipline and control were based on explanation rather than force or coercion

- The extent to which they invited their children to express views about family decisions, in effect valuing the child as a contributor.

Family breakdowns and conflict between parents have also been related to low self-esteem. A person's self-esteem could be harmed due to the lack of concern towards a child or the loss of social support; after all, parents are the primary source of nurture and support for a child. Better communication between child and parent was correlated with better self-esteem.

Gravity of Low Self-Esteem in Men, Women, and Teens

Statistics reveal that the number of people experiencing low self-esteem, especially teenage girls, is skyrocketing. A person with low self-esteem perceives themself as unlovable, incapable, and incompetent, and tends to engage in self-defeating behavior. Keeping these factors in mind, the following collected data represents the low self-esteem in the population of the United States.

In 2014 self-esteem became a National Crisis when *Real Girls, Real Pressure: A National Report on the State of Self-Esteem*, a study conducted with girls between 8 and 17 and commissioned by the Dove Self-Esteem Project, revealed shocking results. The data determined that a majority of the girls (7 in 10) have significantly lower self-esteem, believing that they are not enough in appearance, academics, and relationships. It also revealed that most of these girls are involved in self-destructive behavior that could cause long-lasting damage. Another study reports that at age thirteen, 53% of American girls are "unhappy with their bodies." This grows to 78% by the time girls reach seventeen.

In teenage boys and girls, dissatisfaction with body and physical appearance is concurrent in the research data. For example, among high school students, 15% of guys and 44% of girls seek to lose weight, and 40% of boys seek to increase muscle mass.

Compared to girls with high self-esteem (25%), girls with lower self-esteem (75%) are involved in negative behaviors such as bullying, self-harm, eating disorders, and smoking.

This gender disparity is also visible among adults, with most women having generally low self-esteem than men. According to publish of 2013, *Girls Just Wanna Not Run: The Gender Gap in Young American's Political Ambition,* men were twice as likely as women to report that they "definitely" plan to run for office at some point in the future (14% of men, compared to 7% of women). On the other hand, women were more than 50% more likely than men to assert that they would never run.

How to Raise Self-Esteem?

From most research and evidence, it is apparent that low self-esteem could be raised by changing parents' behavior. This obviously works for children and adolescents. Thus, most of the self-esteem programs that follow research evidence focus on directing parents' behavior. However, studies also indicate what kind of behavior is needed. What actions represent acceptance and approval, including paying attention, taking an interest, listening, encouraging initiative, being fair, and having clear and positive expectations.

Besides changing parents' behavior, low self-esteem can be improved by making other close relations stronger, such as maintaining friendships over time and building new ones. Finding inner skills and capabilities also helps in increasing self-esteem. Finally, as self-esteem is a subjective phenomenon, it can be improved by changing one's subjective perspective about oneself.

Programs like KICK, DARE, GREAT, SMILE, GOA, and others work on causes of low self-esteem and how to conquer them.

Some programs focus on providing specific forms of knowledge, others on developing competencies, or training particular patterns of behavior or modifying existing habits, still others on modifying attitudes or perceptions. There are significant differences in kinds of delivery –individual therapy, self-help, physical exercises, group-based, peer-tutoring, the whole family – in intensity and length. Nevertheless, each of these programs has its strong points and has had some success. It is safe to conclude that despite many impediments, many kinds of interventions can be used to raise self-esteem and break away from the consequences of low self-esteem.

Conclusion
A Dove of Hope

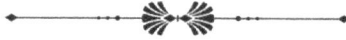

———— ··· ❧ ❧ ··· ————

In fiction and video games, the main character of an adventure symbolically descends into the underworld and confronts dark forces before there can be victory. In my world, at the age of twenty-four, I faced very real horrors and terrors that destroyed my health and peace of mind. I did not have to go far for my serenity to become a nightmare, complete with flames and smoke. Hell was lurking in my own home, it was lingering on the streets I used to travel to work, and it was hiding in the soul of the man who was my husband.

When Hell beckons at one's door, the visit is not limited to a little suffering or adversity. It is the purposeful destruction of everything held dear. It is a test one never forgets. Hell is a trial intended to break us or refine us. It is tribulation meant to make us push ourselves until we reach Heaven.

Enduring physical, mental, and emotional agonies are lessons that call for self-examination. They are experiences that challenge what we think we know, our plentiful lives, the objects we covet, our vanity, and other behavior that stain our morality and character. Hardship forces us to learn about who we are and take control of our actions.

No different than how a savage storm can devastate a mountain forest...hardship can disrupt the lives of good people in unexpected and unimaginable ways. However, storms can also restore the environment by washing away dead leaves, nourishing the soil, and helping plants and trees thrive. Once the turbulence has passed, the sun will shine, the ground will be fertile, the roots will be healthier, and the green will be greener for the storm's energy has passed, and nature will find balance and bounce back stronger than before. People also have the potential to bounce back from setbacks. Do you have the resiliency to bounce back from adversity and conquer another day?

Take the time to find all the positive things in your life, but do not ignore problems and difficulties. No one lives free from strife and worry. If there is something you want to change, something you need to change, start by changing your thinking. The path to happiness is positive thinking; optimism should not be underestimated. Each one of us can build an environment that is rich with love and meaningfulness.

Unfortunately, change is often triggered by some sort of tragedy that encourages transformation. The loss of a loved one, the collapse of a dream, it is these moments of Hell on earth, when we carry the least amount of hope or even lack the willpower to go on living, that motivate us to persevere until we succeed. If only change could be stimulated by a brief discussion with a stranger, or from the power of positive thinking, or from reading a book that casually steers the reader toward the moral and ethical codes of faith.

My personal transformation came when I found myself unable to walk following a devastating automobile accident. The responsibility of caring for my son and then for my brother is what kept me going. The frustration I felt after learning about my husband's infidelity certainly complicated matters. Although I was fortunate to have had friends, my family, and my faith to help me, had my husband stood by me in my time of need, perhaps my rate of recovery would have progressed more swiftly than it did. My support network helped me to avoid dwelling on the negative and look for the positive. They helped me turn chaos into order. Whenever I got close to my breaking point, someone was always there to help me keep reaching for the sky whenever things were dire and bleak.

It is easy to become overwhelmed and resentful when things go wrong. When faced with the insurmountable, it may seem as if there is no way out that you will never be able to overcome the hardships. Before little things become big, it is important to identify and prioritize challenges and determine how to get through each of them, even if it is one inch at a time. If something cannot be repaired, there is no need to dwell on it and waste energy. We must accept what we cannot be changed and adapt to our limitations. Focus on what matters and on what is necessary to move forward.

Believe in yourself. Believe that you are more resilient than you know.

Research: Myth of Mental Health

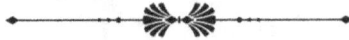

With increasing knowledge and research in psychiatry, psychology, and other mental health-related fields, the world is discovering many ways to tackle and even cure mental health conditions. But there is one impediment that the human race is still laboring to overcome, which is the resistance to seeking mental health care in the first place. There are many reasons as to why this resistance is so hard to break through, one of the most important being the stigma surrounding the mental health conditions, which leads to more myths about treatment.

Mental Health Stigma

A stigma is a complicated construct that associates disgrace to a particular person, place, or thing. It is made of public, self, and structural components.

The thing about stigma is that it not only affects people with mental health illnesses but also impedes its service and support groups. According to Henderson, Evans-Lacko, and Thornicroft (2013), approximately 70% of individuals suffering from a mental health condition do not receive treatment. It is evident that stigma plays a huge role in this percentage; some people just do not have access to treatment, but most do not even try to seek it out. Descriptive studies and epidemiological surveys suggest strong evidence about such factors that increase the probability of treatment avoidance, delays to care, and discontinuation of service use.

Henderson, Evans-Lacko, and Thornicroft (2013) reported that these factors include:

1. Lack of knowledge about the features and treatability of mental illnesses

2. Ignorance about how to access assessment and treatment

3. Prejudice against people who have a mental illness

4. Expectations of discrimination against people who have a diagnosis of mental illness

Myths of Seeking Mental Health Care

Besides the already hard-to-shake stigmas surrounding mental health conditions, there are many myths regarding the help provided by the professionals. The most common of them include;

Myth: Therapy is exclusively for people with severe mental conditions.

This is one of the most common misconceptions. Therapy is not only for extreme illnesses but also for concerns like depression, anxiety, and many other issues. This myth is dangerous as it hinders people with early minor signs of a bigger condition from reaching out for help when that help would be most useful and effective. And even if the condition was not supposed to be severe, the untreated symptoms can grow and do more damage.

Myth: Therapy is a life-long process, and people get stuck in it.

People have this idea that therapy never ends, that once a person starts going to therapy, they are stuck. However, the way therapy works actually depends on a person's condition. Therapists are professionals, and they take the sessions forward so that the person becomes more and more independent (rather than dependent on the therapist). And though the time depends on how soon one reaches whatever goals were set, there is no way a person will be stuck in therapy indefinitely.

Myth: A person should just talk to a friend/family member instead of a professional.

Although it is good to trust your friends and family and share what you are going through, it is also important to remember that they are not professionals. Of course, they can listen, but they cannot indicate any signs of a serious condition, they cannot diagnose you, and most importantly, they usually do not know how to treat a mental health issue. Just as a person with physical illness will not normally go to non-professional for treatment, similarly, a person with psychological concern should not rely on a non-professional for his/her treatment.

Myth: Psychologists just listen to people vent.

Most people believe that counselors and therapists only hear people complain, so it is not intelligent to pay someone for this. This belief is completely false. Even though it is true that a psychologist should be a good listener, this is not where their job ends. Psychologists are trained to unfold the history of a person so they will be able to find different destructive patterns of behavior, various emotional triggers, and most importantly, to find the strengths of a person and help the client use those strengths in self-recovery. All of this is a lot more than just "listening to someone vent."

Myth: Seeking professional help for a mental condition means that the person is labeled forever.

There is indeed a lot of stigma around mental health illness. Still, with increasing knowledge, it is becoming more and more understandable that mental health is a priority and that people suffering are not crazy. On the contrary, people want each other to seek help, which normalizes the practice and lends courage to them and their loved ones to do the same. As studies have shown, according to the National Institute of Mental Health, 1 out of every 5 Americans has a diagnosable mental disorder in their lifetime.

Myth: This is all in our head, and we cannot control it; we are weak.

Another misconception regarding mental health is that there is no actual illness, rather just what we think and feel. Though a person is indeed responsible for their actions and thoughts, they are not responsible for their mental condition. Our thoughts might be abstract, but our brain is a physical organ. It works through its own chemical and hormonal mechanisms. And just like every other organ, we can try our best to keep it function smoothly through ways we are capable of, but sometimes we are not. This is not weakness – rather, it is just accepting our natural human limitations.

Myth: Mental health professionals are there to make money off of people's suffering.

This one is perhaps the most common myth. We often hear that therapy is "too expensive" and that professionals, such as psychologists, psychiatrists, social workers, psychiatric nurses, marriage and family counselors, etc., are just trying to make money off clients' distress. Ryan Howes, Ph.D., and an expert in California notes, "Therapy prices range from free in some community clinics to almost-lawyer hourly rates in the nation's top private practices." Of course, the price ranges vary in different clinics. However, it is important to understand that you are investing in an essential part of your life, something that otherwise might jeopardize your quality of (social, professional, personal) life.

The Gravity of Stigmatization

In 2014, The Lancet Psychiatry published a systematic review that described precisely the growing body of evidence on mental-illness-related stigmatization in health care and its consequences.

According to their review, these consequences included negative stereotypes and attitudes, prognostic negativity, diagnostic overshadowing, insufficient skills of healthcare providers, discriminatory behaviors, and perceptions of unfair treatment among consumers of mental health services. There is a significant mortality gap in high-income countries between people with severe mental illnesses and the general population – 20 years for men and 15 years for women. Many would hold that stigmatization is to blame.

There are two types of stigmas:

1. **Public Stigma** – the assumptions and misconceptions constructed by society.
2. **Self Stigma** – the fear of being stigmatized by society that becomes a barrier in seeking mental health care.

This danger is spreading widely throughout the world, and regrettably, it is has increased despite the increase in knowledge. For example, survey research suggests that a representative 1996 population sample in the U.S. was 2.5 times more likely to endorse the stigma asserting that mental illness was dangerous than a comparable 1950 group, i.e., perceptions that mentally ill people are violent or frightening considerably increased from 1950 to 1996.

Approaches and Interventions

Many research-supported strategies have proven to help change the attitudes of people towards mental health stigmas.

Education

Educational campaigns directed towards correcting misconceptions about mental health conditions and services have proved to be of some help. A brief social media intervention in Canada called *In One Voice* resulted in improved attitudes toward mental health issues and less social distance at a year follow-up. The important part of these educational campaigns is that they need to be professionally designed and organized; campaigns designed to highlight the genetic components of schizophrenia, for example, have sometimes had unintended and stigmatizing consequences. They mistakenly give out the message that recovery is not quite possible and how different the person is from others, whereas it is supposed to take the blame off the person who is suffering.

Contact

One of the main reasons behind myths and stigmas is that people who believe in them have not actually had the chance to experience the process of receiving care from a mental health provider. Therefore, in case of mental illness stigmas, people should be encouraged to contact people suffering from the illness. Online contact, for example, sharing experiences through online posts and video calls, can help initiate the contact and correct the stigmas. In addition, in case of myths about seeking mental health care, people who have reached out to get treatment should be encouraged to share their experience with other people; this will help counterbalance the misconceptions and give hope to the people who are afraid to seek help.

Protest and Policy Change

By advocating human rights, awareness can be spread across the globe leading to positive changes regarding policies concerning mental health. This can help pressure the government to protect people with mental health issues and make resources available for treatment. Policy changes have proved successful before decreasing stigmas, beginning with the prohibition of discrimination by race, color, religion, and national origin in all public accommodations in The Civil Rights Act of 1964. As a result, there was a considerable drop in the mortality rate of black Americans in the 1960s and 1970s, which can be linked to legislation that prohibited racial discrimination in Medicare payments for hospital-based care.

Resources

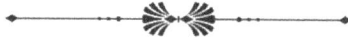

Jerry Healing Hands, Inc.
Bereavement Support Program- call 954-451-0365

Managed and directed by Kettlyne St. Cyr, Nurse Practitioner, a seasoned behavioral health professional. Our mission is to help people work through their personal loss and grief. Our services are currently held in easily accessible locations in Miami-Dade County. We offer twelve-week group programs to the participants.

Jerry Healing Hands, Inc. also offers medication management and group therapy sessions for a variety of mental health needs.

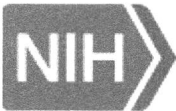

National Institute
of Mental Health

Call 911 if you or someone you know is in immediate danger or go to the nearest emergency room.

The Recovery Village Miami at Baptist Health Drug and Alcohol Rehab-Mental Health
8585 Sunset Dr. Suite 202 Miami, FL 33143
Call 786-780-1408

National Suicide Prevention Lifeline
Call 1-800-273-TALK (8255); En español 1-888-628-9454
The Lifeline is a free, confidential crisis hotline that is available to everyone 24 hours a day, seven days a week. The Lifeline connects callers to the nearest crisis center in the Lifeline national network. These centers provide crisis counseling and mental health referrals. People who are deaf, hard of hearing, or have hearing loss can contact the Lifeline via TTY at 1-800-799-4889.

Crisis Text Line
Text "HELLO" to 741741
The Crisis Text hotline is available 24 hours a day, seven days a week throughout the U.S. The Crisis Text Line serves anyone in any type of crisis, connecting them with a crisis counselor who can provide support and information.

Veterans Crisis Line
Call 1-800-273-TALK (8255) and press 1 or text to 838255
The Veterans Crisis Line is a free, confidential resource that connects veterans 24 hours a day, seven days a week, with a trained responder. The service is available to all veterans, even if they are not registered with the VA or enrolled in VA healthcare. People who are deaf, hard of hearing, or have hearing loss can call 1-800-799-4889.

Disaster Distress Helpline
Call or text 1-800-985-5990
The disaster distress helpline provides immediate crisis counseling for people who are experiencing emotional distress related to any natural or human-caused disaster. The helpline is free, multilingual, confidential, and available 24 hours a day, seven days a week.

Homeless Trust
1-877-994-4357
http://homelesstrust.org/

National Institute on Drug Abuse Hotline
(800) 662-4357

Poison Control
(800) 222-1222

SAMHSA's Toll-Free Treatment Referral Helpline:
1-800-662-HELP (4357)

Children's Bereavement
www.ChildBereavement.org
1-888-988-5438

The HELPline- Miami Dade
(305) 358-HELP (4357)
(305) 358-2477 TDD/TTY

The Teen Link Line
(305) 377-TEEN (8336)
80 Taped Messages for Teens

Teen Talk Line
(305) 377-TALK (8255)
To Speak to a Counselor

Children & Youth Behavioral Hotline
(305) 358-HELP (4357)

First Call For Help - Broward County
24-Hour Helplines - Dial 211
(954) 537-0211

First Call for Seniors
(954) 390-0485

Teen Hotline
(954) 567-TEEN
(954) 567-8336

Phone Friend for Kids up to 13
(954) 390-0486

National Alliance Mental Illness- Miami Dade County
CALL 305-665-2540
https://Namimiami.org

References

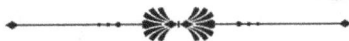

#BeThere To Help Prevent Suicide. Centers for Disease Control. Retrieved from https://www.cdc.gov/injury/features/be-there-prevent-suicide/index.html

11 Facts About Teens and Self Esteem. (2020). DoSomething.Org. https://www.dosomething.org/us/facts/11-facts-about-teens-and-self-esteem

Abdel-Khalek, A. M. (2016, October 1). Introduction to the Psychology of self-esteem. ResearchGate. https://www.researchgate.net/publication/311440256_Introduction_to_the_Psychology_of_self-esteem

Ahmadimanesh, M., Abbaszadegan, M., Morshedi Rad, D., Moallem, S., Mohammadpour, A., & Ghahremani, M. et al. (2019). Effects of selective serotonin reuptake inhibitors on DNA damage in patients with depression. Journal Of Psychopharmacology, 33(11), 1364-1376. https://doi.org/10.1177/0269881119874461

American Psychiatric Association. (2020, October). What Is Depression? Web Starter Kit. https://www.psychiatry.org/patients-families/depression/what-is-depression

American Public Health Association (APHA) Publications. https://ajph.aphapublications.org/action/cookieAbsent

An American Addiction Centers Recourse. (2020). Treatment: When to Seek Professional Help and Where to Find Help for Major Depression. Mentalhelp.Net. https://www.mentalhelp.net/depression/when-to-seek-professional-help/

Andrade, L. (2018). On the death of mi madre, hauntings, and ethnic mourning. Text And Performance Quarterly, 38(3), 136-152. https://doi.org/10.1080/10462937.2018.1468572

Andreassen CS, Pallesen S, Griffiths MD. The relationship between addictive use of social media, narcissism, and self-esteem: Findings from a large national survey. Addict Behav. 2017 Jan;64:287-293. DOI: https://doi.org/10.1016/j.addbeh.2016.03.006

Apelian, E., & Nesteruk, O. (2017). REFLECTIONS OF YOUNG ADULTS ON THE LOSS OF A PARENT IN ADOLESCENCE. International Journal Of Child, Youth And Family Studies, 8(3/4), 79. https://doi.org/10.18357/ijcyfs83/4201718002

Approaches to Reducing Stigma - Ending Discrimination Against People with Mental and Substance Use Disorders. NCBI Bookshelf. https://www.ncbi.nlm.nih.gov/books/NBK384914/

Bailey, K., & Gammage, K. (2019). Applying Action Research in a Mixed Methods Positive Body Image Program Assessment With Older Adults and People With Physical Disability and Chronic Illness. Journal Of Mixed Methods Research, 14(2), 248-267. https://doi.org/10.1177/1558689819871814

Barbano, A., der Mei, W., deRoon ‑ Cassini, T., Grauer, E., Lowe, S., & Matsuoka, Y. et al. (2019). Differentiating PTSD from anxiety and depression: Lessons from the ICD ‑ 11 PTSD diagnostic criteria. Depression And Anxiety, 36(6), 490-498. https://doi.org/10.1002/da.22881

Bartone, P., Bartone, J., Violanti, J., & Gileno, Z. (2017). Peer Support Services for Bereaved Survivors: A Systematic Review. OMEGA - Journal Of Death And Dying, 80(1), 137-166. https://doi.org/10.1177/0030222817728204

Baumeister, R. F., & Leary, M. R. (1995). The need to belong: Desire for interpersonal attachments as a fundamental human motivation. Psychological Bulletin, 117(3), 497–529. https://pubmed.ncbi.nlm.nih.gov/7777651/

Baxter, A. J., Tweed, E. J., & Vittal, S. (2018). Effects of Housing First approaches on health and well-being of adults who are homeless or at risk of homelessness: systematic review and meta-analysis of randomized controlled trials | IGH Hub. Ruff Institute of Global Homelessness. https://ighhub.org/resource/effects-housing-first-approaches-health-and-well-being-adults-who-are-homeless-or-risk

Behavioral & Mental Health (IPD). (2020, August 7). Debunking 8 Myths About Seeking Mental

Benjamin, E., Muntner, P., Alonso, A., Bittencourt, M., Callaway, C., & Carson, A. et al. (2019). Heart Disease and Stroke Statistics—2019 Update: A Report From the American Heart Association. Circulation, 139(10). https://doi.org/10.1161/cir.0000000000000659

Bruce, D. F. (2008, May 22). Types of Depression. WebMD. https://www.webmd.com/depression/guide/depression-types

Cameron, J., & Granger, S. (2016). Self-Esteem and Belongingness. Encyclopedia of Personality and Individual Differences, 1–3. https://doi.org/10.1007/978-3-319-28099-8_1170-1

Carr, D. (2020). Psychological Resilience in the Face of Later-Life Spousal Bereavement. Resilience And Aging, 157-174. https://doi.org/10.1007/978-3-030-57089-7_8

Centre for Addiction and Mental Health (CAMH). (2020). Addressing Stigma. CAMH. https://www.camh.ca/en/driving-change/addressing-stigma

Choi, J., Kaghazchi, A., Dickerson, K., Tennakoon, L., Spain, D., & Forrester, J. (2021). Heterogeneity in managing rib fractures across non-trauma and level I, II, and III trauma centers. The American Journal Of Surgery. https://doi.org/10.1016/j.amjsurg.2021.02.013

Claire Henderson, Sara Evans-Lacko, and Graham Thornicroft, 2013:

CMHC Self Esteem. (2021). UT Counseling and Mental Health Center. https://cmhc.utexas.edu/selfesteem.html

Coelho, A., de Brito, M., & Barbosa, A. (2018). Caregiver anticipatory grief: phenomenology, assessment and clinical interventions. Current Opinion In Supportive & Palliative Care, 12(1), 52-57. https://doi.org/10.1097/spc.0000000000000321

Committee on the Science of Changing Behavioral Health Social Norms. (2016, August 3).

Contractor, A., Greene, T., Dolan, M., & Elhai, J. (2018). Relations between PTSD and depression symptom clusters in samples differentiated by PTSD diagnostic status. Journal Of Anxiety Disorders, 59, 17-26. https://doi.org/10.1016/j.janxdis.2018.08.004

Corrigan, P. W. Druss, B. G. Perlick, D. A. (2014, September). The Impact of Mental Illness

Cozza, S., Fisher, J., Zhou, J., Harrington-LaMorie, J., La Flair, L., Fullerton, C., & Ursano, R. (2017). Bereaved Military Dependent Spouses and Children: Those Left Behind in a Decade of War (2001–2011). Military Medicine, 182(3), e1684-e1690. https://doi.org/10.7205/milmed-d-16-00101

Dahlby, L., & Kerr, T. (2020). PTSD and opioid use: implications for intervention and policy. Substance Abuse Treatment, Prevention, And Policy, 15(1). https://doi.org/10.1186/s13011-020-00264-8

Dantchev, S., Zammit, S., & Wolke, D. (2018). Sibling bullying in middle childhood and psychotic disorder at 18 years: a prospective cohort study. Psychological Medicine, 48(14), 2321-2328. https://doi.org/10.1017/s0033291717003841

Dauphin, V. (2020). A critique of the American Psychological Association Clinical Practice Guideline for the Treatment of Posttraumatic Stress Disorder (PTSD) in Adults. Psychoanalytic Psychology, 37(2), 117-127. https://doi.org/10.1037/pap0000253

Dawson, B. (2020, February 18). The State of America's Children 2020 - Housing and Homelessness — Children's Defense Fund. Children's Defense Fund. https://www.childrensdefense.org/policy/resources/soac-2020-housing/

De Freitas, C., Jordan, H., & Hughes, E. (2018). Body image diversity in the media: A content analysis of women's fashion magazines. Health Promotion Journal Of Australia, 29(3), 251-256. https://doi.org/10.1002/hpja.21

Degenhardt, L., Saha, S., Lim, C., Aguilar-Gaxiola, S., Al-Hamzawi, A., & Alonso, J. et al. (2018). The associations between psychotic experiences and substance use and substance use disorders: findings from the World Health Organization World Mental Health surveys. Addiction, 113(5), 924-934. https://doi.org/10.1111/add.14145

Demographic Data Project: Gender and Individual Homelessness. (2019, September 30). National Alliance to End Homelessness. https://endhomelessness.org/demographic-data-project-gender-and-individual-homelessness/

Depression: Supporting a family member or friend. (2018, November 28). Mayo Clinic. https://www.mayoclinic.org/diseases-conditions/depression/in-depth/depression/art-20045943

Devrim, A., Bilgic, P., & Hongu, N. (2018). Is There Any Relationship Between Body Image Perception, Eating Disorders, and Muscle Dysmorphic Disorders in Male Bodybuilders? American Journal Of Men's Health, 12(5), 1746-1758. https://doi.org/10.1177/1557988318786868

Dye, H. (2018). The impact and long-term effects of childhood trauma. Journal Of Human Behavior In The Social Environment, 28(3), 381-392. https://doi.org/10.1080/10911359.2018.1435328

Eisma, M., Lenferink, L., Chow, A., Chan, C., & Li, J. (2019). Complicated grief and post-traumatic stress symptom profiles in bereaved earthquake survivors: a latent class analysis. European Journal Of Psychotraumatology, 10(1), 1558707. https://doi.org/10.1080/20008198.2018.1558707

Emler, N. (2001, January 1). Self-esteem: The costs and causes of low self-worth. ResearchGate. https://www.researchgate.net/publication/30530126_Self_esteem_T he_costs_and_causes_of_low_self_worth

Felsen, I. (2018). Parental trauma and adult sibling relationships in Holocaust-survivor families. Psychoanalytic Psychology, 35(4), 433-445. https://doi.org/10.1037/pap0000196

Foa, E., Asnaani, A., Zang, Y., Capaldi, S., & Yeh, R. (2017). Psychometrics of the Child PTSD Symptom Scale for DSM-5 for Trauma-Exposed Children and Adolescents. Journal Of Clinical Child & Adolescent Psychology, 47(1), 38-46. https://doi.org/10.1080/15374416.2017.1350962

Freire, R., Cabrera-Abreu, C., & Milev, R. (2020). Neurostimulation in Anxiety Disorders, Post-traumatic Stress Disorder, and Obsessive-Compulsive Disorder. Advances In Experimental Medicine And Biology, 331-346. https://doi.org/10.1007/978-981-32-9705-0_18

Frequently Asked Questions about Depression. (2020, February 26). Brain & Behavior Research Foundation. https://www.bbrfoundation.org/faq/frequently-asked-questions-about-depression?gclid=Cj0KCQjw9YWDBhDyARIsADt6sGY-pNPfeiho3L2jFOdIaq5XXlczVb7v4bGnNTCzLdG1urfmvxi1cgAa AqLCEALw_wcB

Fung, X., Pakpour, A., Wu, Y., Fan, C., Lin, C., & Tsang, H. (2019). Psychosocial Variables Related to Weight-Related Self-Stigma in Physical Activity among Young Adults across Weight Status. International Journal Of Environmental Research And Public Health, 17(1), 64. https://doi.org/10.3390/ijerph17010064

Gentile, A., Servidio, R., Caci, B., & Boca, S. (2018). Social stigma and self-esteem as mediators of the relationship between Body Mass Index and Internet addiction disorder. An exploratory study. Current Psychology, 40(3), 1262-1270. https://doi.org/10.1007/s12144-018-0054-x

Giraldo-O'Meara, M., & Belloch, A. (2018). Escalation from normal appearance-related intrusive cognitions to clinical preoccupations in Body Dysmorphic Disorder: A cross-sectional study. Psychiatry Research, 265, 137-143. https://doi.org/10.1016/j.psychres.2018.04.047

Girls Just Wanna Not Run The Gender Gap in Young Americans' Political Ambition. (2013, March). Jennifer L. Lawless, Richard L. Fox. https://www.american.edu/spa/wpi/upload/girls-just-wanna-not-run_policy-report.pdf

GoodTherapy Editor Team. (2019, July 3). Rejection. GoodTherapy. https://www.goodtherapy.org/learn-about-therapy/issues/rejection

Gorrell, S., & Murray, S. (2019). Eating Disorders in Males. Child And Adolescent Psychiatric Clinics Of North America, 28(4), 641-651. https://doi.org/10.1016/j.chc.2019.05.012

Greenberg, J., Weingarden, H., & Wilhelm, S. (2019). A Practical Guide to Managing Body Dysmorphic Disorder in the Cosmetic Surgery Setting. JAMA Facial Plastic Surgery, 21(3), 181-182. https://doi.org/10.1001/jamafacial.2018.1840

Grohol, J. M. (1998, February). Top 10 Myths About Mental Health. Counseling and

Groß, J., Blank, H., & Bayen, U. (2017). Hindsight Bias in Depression. Clinical Psychological Science, 5(5), 771-788. https://doi.org/10.1177/2167702617712262

Health Therapy. DuPage Medical Group. https://www.dupagemedicalgroup.com/health-topic/debunking-8-myths-about-seeking-mental-health-therapy

Henderson, C. (2013, May). Mental Illness Stigma, Help Seeking, and Public Health Programs.

Homelessness and Mental Illness: A Challenge to Our Society. (2018, November 19). Brain & Behavior Research Foundation. https://www.bbrfoundation.org/blog/homelessness-and-mental-illness-challenge-our-society

Hope for Depression. (2021, January 25). Facts about Depression | Hope for Depression. https://www.hopefordepression.org/depression-facts/?gclid=Cj0KCQjw9YWDBhDyARIsADt6sGY_dQBZyHIOm bkrVD0pWqQeUALt-HSarUwR1_DstgCpPxJCMpQ0rEMaAgAXEALw_wcB

Hübel, C., Abdulkadir, M., Herle, M., Loos, R., Breen, G., Bulik, C., & Micali, N. (2021). One size does not fit all. Genomics differentiates among anorexia nervosa, bulimia nervosa, and binge - eating disorder. International Journal Of Eating Disorders. https://doi.org/10.1002/eat.23481

Hutson, S., Hall, J., & Pack, F. (2015). Survivor Guilt. Advances In Nursing Science, 38(1), 20-33. https://doi.org/10.1097/ans.0000000000000058

Impact on Mental Health | IGH Hub. (2020). Ruff Institute of Global Homelessness. https://ighhub.org/understanding-homelessness/impact-mental-health

Invisible Depression. (2020, October 16). GraceMed Health Clinic. https://gracemed.org/hidden-depression

James, W. (1890). The Principles of Psychology. Google Books. https://books.google.com.pk/books/about/The_Principles_of_Psychology.html?id=JLcAAAAMAAJ&printsec=frontcover&source=kp_read_button&redir_esc=y#v=onepage&q&f=false

Jaremka, L. M., Ackerman, J. M., Gawronski, B., Rule, N. O., Sweeny, K., Tropp, L. R., Metz, M. A., Molina, L., Ryan, W. S., & Vick, S. B. (2020). Common Academic Experiences No One Talks About: Repeated Rejection, Impostor Syndrome, and Burnout. Perspectives on Psychological Science, 15(3), 519–543. https://doi.org/10.1177/1745691619898848

Kantha, K., Rani, M.U, Parameswaran, A., Indira, A. (2016). The knowledge regarding eating disorders among adolescent girls. International Journal of Applied Research; 2(5): 864-866

Kashdan, T. B. (2014, March 4). Who Is Most Vulnerable to Social Rejection? The Toxic Combination of Low Self-Esteem and Lack of Negative Emotion Differentiation on Neural Responses to Rejection. Plosone. https://journals.plos.org/plosone/article?id=10.1371/journal.pone.0090651

Kling, K. C., Hyde, J. S., Showers, C. J., & Buswell, B. N. (1999). Gender differences in self-esteem: A meta-analysis. Psychological

Bulletin, 125(4), 470–500. https://doi.org/10.1037/0033-2909.125.4.470

Knaak S, Patten S, Ungar T. (2015) Mental illness stigma as a quality of care problem.

Kostecka, B., Kordyńska, K., Murawiec, S., & Kucharska, K. (2019). Distorted body image in women and men suffering from Anorexia Nervosa – a literature review. Archives Of Psychiatry And Psychotherapy, 21(1), 13-21. https://doi.org/10.12740/app/102833

Krediet, E., Bostoen, T., Breeksema, J., van Schagen, A., Passie, T., & Vermetten, E. (2020). Reviewing the Potential of Psychedelics for the Treatment of PTSD. International Journal Of Neuropsychopharmacology, 23(6), 385-400. https://doi.org/10.1093/ijnp/pyaa018

Leary, M. R. (2015, December 1). Emotional responses to interpersonal rejection. PubMed Central (PMC). https://www.ncbi.nlm.nih.gov/pmc/articles/PMC4734881/

Leary, M. R., Schreindorfer, L. S., & Haupt, A. L. (1995). The Role of Low Self-Esteem in Emotional and Behavioral Problems: Why is Low Self-Esteem Dysfunctional? Journal of Social and Clinical Psychology, 14(3), 297–314. https://doi.org/10.1521/jscp.1995.14.3.297

Lehigh Center for Clinical Research. (2020). The Importance Of Seeking Mental Health Treatment. Lehigh Center. https://www.lehighcenter.com/the-importance-of-seeking-mental-health-treatment/

LeRoy, A., Gabert, T., Garcini, L., Murdock, K., Heijnen, C., & Fagundes, C. (2020). Attachment orientations and loss adjustment among bereaved spouses. Psychoneuroendocrinology, 112, 104401. https://doi.org/10.1016/j.psyneuen.2019.104401

Livingston, N., Lee, D., Mahoney, C., Farmer, S., Cole, T., Marx, B., & Keane, T. (2021). Longitudinal assessment of PTSD and illicit drug use among male and female OEF-OIF veterans. Addictive Behaviors, 118, 106870. https://doi.org/10.1016/j.addbeh.2021.106870

López - Castro, T., Saraiya, T., Zumberg - Smith, K., & Dambreville, N. (2019). Association Between Shame and Posttraumatic Stress Disorder: A Meta - Analysis. Journal Of Traumatic Stress, 32(4), 484-495. https://doi.org/10.1002/jts.22411

Luck, T., & Luck-Sikorski, C. (2020). Feelings of guilt in the general adult population: prevalence, intensity and association with depression. Psychology, Health & Medicine, 1-11. https://doi.org/10.1080/13548506.2020.1859558

Manaf, N. (2016). The Prevalence and Inter-Relationship of Negative Body Image Perception, Depression and Susceptibility to Eating Disorders among Female Medical Undergraduate Students. JOURNAL OF CLINICAL AND DIAGNOSTIC RESEARCH. https://doi.org/10.7860/jcdr/2016/16678.7341

Mastro, D., & Figueroa-Caballero, A. (2018). Measuring Extremes: A Quantitative Content Analysis of Prime Time TV Depictions of Body Type. Journal Of Broadcasting & Electronic Media, 62(2), 320-336. https://doi.org/10.1080/08838151.2018.1451853

Mcleod, S. (2012). Low Self Esteem. Simply Psychology. https://www.simplypsychology.org/self-esteem.html

McMillan, K., Asmundson, G., & Sareen, J. (2017). Comorbid PTSD and Social Anxiety Disorder. Journal Of Nervous & Mental Disease, 205(9), 732-737. https://doi.org/10.1097/nmd.0000000000000704

Mental Illness Stigma, Help Seeking, and Public Health Programs. American Journal of Public Health 103, 777_780, https://doi.org/10.2105/AJPH.2012.301056

Miao, X., Chen, Q., Wei, K., Tao, K., & Lu, Z. (2018). Posttraumatic stress disorder: from diagnosis to prevention. Military Medical Research, 5(1). https://doi.org/10.1186/s40779-018-0179-0

Miron, O., Yu, K., Wilf-Miron, R., & Kohane, I. (2019). Suicide Rates Among Adolescents and Young Adults in the United States, 2000-2017. JAMA, 321(23), 2362. https://doi.org/10.1001/jama.2019.5054

Moreno-Domínguez, S., Servián-Franco, F., Reyes del Paso, G., & Cepeda-Benito, A. (2018). Images of Thin and Plus-Size Models Produce Opposite Effects on Women's Body Image, Body Dissatisfaction, and Anxiety. Sex Roles, 80(9-10), 607-616. https://doi.org/10.1007/s11199-018-0951-3

Morin, A. (2021, February). Could You Have Smiling Depression? Verywell Mind. https://www.verywellmind.com/what-is-smiling-depression-4775918#risk-of-suicide

Morris, A. M., & Katzman, D. K. (2003). The impact of the media on eating disorders in children and adolescents. Paediatrics & child health, 8(5), 287–289. https://doi.org/10.1093/pch/8.5.287

Mountford, V., & Koskina, A. (2015). Body Image. Encyclopedia Of Feeding And Eating Disorders, 1-5. https://doi.org/10.1007/978-981-287-087-2_74-1

Murnen, S., & Smolak, L. (2019). The Cash effect: Shaping the research conversation on body image and eating disorders. Body Image, 31, 288-293. https://doi.org/10.1016/j.bodyim.2019.01.001

Murray, H. (2018). Survivor Guilt in a Posttraumatic Stress Disorder Clinic Sample. Journal Of Loss And Trauma, 23(7), 600-607. https://doi.org/10.1080/15325024.2018.1507965

National Center on Family Homelessness. (2018, September 27). American Institutes for Research. https://www.air.org/center/national-center-family-homelessness#:%7E:text=A%20staggering%202.5%20million%20children,children%20in%20the%20United%20States.

National Institute of Mental Health. (2019, February 1). NIMH » Major Depression. NIMH. https://www.nimh.nih.gov/health/statistics/major-depression.shtml

Neimeyer, R. (2019). Meaning reconstruction in bereavement: Development of a research program. Death Studies, 43(2), 79-91. https://doi.org/10.1080/07481187.2018.1456620

Nicholson, J. (2020, September 29). Understanding and Dealing With Interpersonal Rejection. Psychology Today. https://www.psychologytoday.com/intl/blog/the-attraction-doctor/202009/understanding-and-dealing-interpersonal-rejection

Norman, S., Haller, M., Hamblen, J., Southwick, S., & Pietrzak, R. (2018). The burden of co-occurring alcohol use disorder and PTSD in U.S. Military veterans: Comorbidities, functioning, and suicidality. Psychology Of Addictive Behaviors, 32(2), 224-229. https://doi.org/10.1037/adb0000348

Orth, U., Robins, R. W., & Meier, L. L. (2009). Disentangling the effects of low self-esteem and stressful events on depression: Findings from three longitudinal studies. Journal of Personality and Social Psychology, 97(2), 307–321. https://doi.org/10.1037/a0015645

Ortiz-Ospina, E. (2017, February 16). Homelessness. Our World in Data. https://ourworldindata.org/homelessness

Perng, A., & Renz, S. (2018). Identifying and Treating Complicated Grief in Older Adults. The Journal For Nurse Practitioners, 14(4), 289-295. https://doi.org/10.1016/j.nurpra.2017.12.001

Providing support for those experiencing homelessness | Volunteers of America. (2020). Volunteers of America: National. https://www.voa.org/homeless-people

Psychological Services. https://mhs.tcnj.edu/top-10-myths-about-mental-health/

Radziwiłłowicz, W., & Lewandowska, M. (2017). From Traumatic Events and Dissociation to Body Image and Depression Symptoms – in Search of Self-Destruction Syndrome in Adolescents who Engage in Nonsuicidal Self-Injury. Psychiatria Polska, 51(2), 283-301. https://doi.org/10.12740/pp/63801

Rafferty, Y., & Shinn, M. (1991). The impact of homelessness on children. American Psychologist, 46(11), 1170–1179. https://doi.org/10.1037/0003-066X.46.11.1170

Retrieved from http://www.thelancet.com/journals/lanpsy/issue/current

Richards, A., Kanady, J., & Neylan, T. (2019). Sleep disturbance in PTSD and other anxiety-related disorders: an updated review of clinical features, physiological characteristics, and psychological and neurobiological mechanisms. Neuropsychopharmacology, 45(1), 55-73. https://doi.org/10.1038/s41386-019-0486-5

Robbins-Welty, G., Stahl, S., & Reynolds, C. (2017). Grief Reactions in the Elderly. Clinical Handbook Of Bereavement And Grief Reactions, 103-137. https://doi.org/10.1007/978-3-319-65241-2_6

Rüsch, N. (2020, April). Mental illness stigma: Concepts, consequences, and initiatives to reduce stigma | European

Psychiatry. Cambridge Core.
https://www.cambridge.org/core/journals/european-psychiatry/article/mental-illness-stigma-concepts-consequences-and-initiatives-to-reduce-stigma/3AE7283F0F35980994B4BD71E92C3C08

Ryding, F., & Kuss, D. (2020). The use of social networking sites, body image dissatisfaction, and body dysmorphic disorder: A systematic review of psychological research. Psychology Of Popular Media, 9(4), 412-435. https://doi.org/10.1037/ppm0000264

Sandgren, S., & Lavallee, D. (2018). Muscle Dysmorphia Research Neglects DSM-5 Diagnostic Criteria. Journal Of Loss And Trauma, 23(3), 211-243. https://doi.org/10.1080/15325024.2018.1428484

Sangalang, C., Becerra, D., Mitchell, F., Lechuga-Peña, S., Lopez, K., & Kim, I. (2018). Trauma, Post-Migration Stress, and Mental Health: A Comparative Analysis of Refugees and Immigrants in the United States. Journal Of Immigrant And Minority Health, 21(5), 909-919. https://doi.org/10.1007/s10903-018-0826-2

Savage, S. (2008, October 7). New National Report Reveals the High Price of Low Self-Esteem. Redorbit. https://www.redorbit.com/news/health/1580382/new_national_report_reveals_the_high_price_of_low_selfesteem/

Schmitz, C. L., Wagner, J. D., & Menke, E. M. (1995). Homelessness as one component of housing instability and its impact on the development of children in poverty. Journal of Social Distress & the Homeless, 4(4), 301–317. https://doi.org/10.1007/BF02087868

Scocco, P., Preti, A., Totaro, S., Corrigan, P., & Castriotta, C. (2019). Stigma, grief and depressive symptoms in help-seeking people bereaved through suicide. Journal Of Affective Disorders, 244, 223-230. https://doi.org/10.1016/j.jad.2018.10.098

Self-Esteem Statistics on Teens. (2020).
https://static1.squarespace.com/static/58eece343e00beca82f547b5/t/
594ebf79b6ac5081d7fa9895/1498333050084/InfographicSources.pd
f

Sheppard, S. (2020, July 2). The Correlation Between Homelessness
and Mental Health. Verywell Mind.
https://www.verywellmind.com/homelessness-impacts-mental-
health-4783106

Smid, G., Groen, S., de la Rie, S., Kooper, S., & Boelen, P. (2018).
Toward Cultural Assessment of Grief and Grief-Related
Psychopathology. Psychiatric Services, 69(10), 1050-1052.
https://doi.org/10.1176/appi.ps.201700422

Smith, M. (2020). Who's to blame? Rational and irrational
reflections on responsibility following the suicide of a service user.
Journal Of Social Work Practice, 1-12.
https://doi.org/10.1080/02650533.2020.1737517

Social rejection | Psychology Wiki | Fandom. (2019). Psychology
Wiki. https://psychology.wikia.org/wiki/Social_rejection

State of Homelessness: 2020 Edition. (2021, February 9). National
Alliance to End Homelessness.
https://endhomelessness.org/homelessness-in-
america/homelessness-statistics/state-of-homelessness-2020/

Statistics on Girls & Women's Self Esteem, Pressures & Leadership
Heart of Leadership: Lead. Your World. (2015, June 5). Heart of
Leadership. https://heartofleadership.org/statistics/

Steenkamp, M., Schlenger, W., Corry, N., Henn-Haase, C., Qian,
M., & Li, M. et al. (2017). Predictors of PTSD 40 years after
combat: Findings from the National Vietnam Veterans longitudinal
study. Depression And Anxiety, 34(8), 711-722.
https://doi.org/10.1002/da.22628

Stein, A., Dalton, L., Rapa, E., Bluebond-Langner, M., Hanington, L., & Stein, K. et al. (2019). Communication with children and adolescents about the diagnosis of their own life-threatening condition. The Lancet, 393(10176), 1150-1163. https://doi.org/10.1016/s0140-6736(18)33201-x

Stevenson, M., Achille, M., Liben, S., Proulx, M., Humbert, N., & Petti, A. et al. (2016). Understanding How Bereaved Parents Cope With Their Grief to Inform the Services Provided to Them. Qualitative Health Research, 27(5), 649-664. https://doi.org/10.1177/1049732315622189

Stigma on Seeking and Participating in Mental Health Care. SAGE Journals. https://journals.sagepub.com/action/cookieAbsent

Strudwicke, L. (2000). Sense of Belonging and Self-Esteem: What are the Implications for Educational Outcomes of Secondary School Students? : A Literature Review. Research Online. https://ro.ecu.edu.au/theses_hons/867/

Szczotka, J., & Majchrowicz, B. (2018). Schizophrenia as a disorder of embodied self. Psychiatria Polska, 52(2), 199-215. https://doi.org/10.12740/pp/67276

The Lancet Psychiatry; 2: 863-64

Thompson, J., & Schaefer, L. (2019). Thomas F. Cash: A multidimensional innovator in the measurement of body image; Some lessons learned and some lessons for the future of the field. Body Image, 31, 198-203. https://doi.org/10.1016/j.bodyim.2019.08.006

Trevino, K., Litz, B., Papa, A., Maciejewski, P., Lichtenthal, W., Healy, C., & Prigerson, H. (2018). Bereavement Challenges and Their Relationship to Physical and Psychological Adjustment to Loss. Journal Of Palliative Medicine, 21(4), 479-488. https://doi.org/10.1089/jpm.2017.0386

Tyler, K. A., & Malender, L. A. (2015). Child Abuse, Street Victimization, and Substance use Among Homeless Young Adults | IGH Hub. Ruff Institute of Global Homelessness. https://ighhub.org/resource/child-abuse-street-victimization-and-substance-use-among-homeless-young-adults-0

Wang, Y., & Ollendick, T. H. (2001). A cross-cultural and developmental analysis of self-esteem in Chinese and Western children. Clinical Child and Family Psychology Review, 4(3), 253–271. https://doi.org/10.1023/A:1017551215413

Watkins, E., & Roberts, H. (2020). Reflecting on rumination: Consequences, causes, mechanisms and treatment of rumination. Behaviour Research And Therapy, 127, 103573. https://doi.org/10.1016/j.brat.2020.103573

Watson, C., & Ban, S. (2021). Body dysmorphic disorder in children and young people. British Journal Of Nursing, 30(3), 160-164. https://doi.org/10.12968/bjon.2021.30.3.160

Weir, K. (2012). The pain of social rejection. American Psychological Association. https://www.apa.org/monitor/2012/04/rejection

What is Homelessness? | The Homeless Hub. (2019). Homeless Hub. https://homelesshub.ca/resource/what-homelessness

When Sadness Becomes Clinical Depression: Signs to Look For. (2008, June 4). WebMD. https://www.webmd.com/depression/guide/what-is-depression

When to Seek Professional Help for Anxiety and Depression - More Than Just the "Blues" | Prospect Medical Systems. (2020). Prospect Medical. https://www.prospectmedical.com/resources/wellness-center/when-seek-professional-help-anxiety-and-depression-more-just-blues

Why Self-Esteem is Important and Its Dimensions. (2020). MentalHelp.Net. https://www.mentalhelp.net/self-esteem/why-its-important/

Zakarian, R., McDevitt-Murphy, M., Bellet, B., Neimeyer, R., & Burke, L. (2019). Relations Among Meaning Making, PTSD, and Complicated Grief Following Homicide Loss. Journal Of Loss And Trauma, 24(3), 279-291. https://doi.org/10.1080/15325024.2019.1565111